Managing Your Child's Diabetes

Managing Your Child's Diabetes

Robert Wood Johnson IV,
Sale Johnson, Casey Johnson,
and Susan Kleinman

MasterMedia Limited, *New York*

Library of Congress Cataloging-in-Publication Data

Managing your child's diabetes / Robert Wood Johnson IV . . . [et al.].

        p.   cm.
Previously published book: New York: MasterMedia, 1992.
    Includes index.
    ISBN 1–57101–025–4
    1. Diabetes in children—Popular works.   2. Diabetes in children—Patients—Home care.   I. Johnson, Robert Wood.
  RJ420.D5M36   1994
  618.92′462—dc20   *94-3508*
                                                           CIP

Designed by Jacqueline Schuman
Production services by Martin Cook Associates, Ltd.
Manufactured in the United States of America

10 9 8 7 6 5 4 3 2 1

A C K N O W L E D G M E N T S

The authors would like to thank the following people for their help in this project:

Susan Stautberg, our publisher and friend, for believing in our idea and helping us turn it into a reality.

Ken Farber, Karen Brownlee, and the staff at the Juvenile Diabetes Foundation International (JDF), for all the help, information, and assistance they gave us. We could not have completed this book without them.

Fredda Ginsberg-Fellner, M.D.; Paula Liguori, R.N., C.D.E.; and the staff of the Young People's Diabetes Treatment Unit at the Mount Sinai Medical Center in New York for their help and advice.

The experts who shared their knowledge with us: Penelope Buschman, R.N., C.E., Assistant Professor of Nursing at the Columbia University School of Nursing in New York; Barbara Davis; Dr. Maryann Feldstein; Bernard Kleinman, C.P.A., A.P.F.S.; Nancy Sander; Lynne Scott, M.A., R.D./ L.D.; and Shirley Swope.

Neil Burmeister, Chaim Jaroslawicz, and Eunice Kleinman for helping in so many ways.

And last but not least, the parents who shared their experiences and insights with us: Thomas Borger, Susan Briston, Carol Brownstein, Sandra Gandy, LuNell and Joseph Garza, Ms. Goldsmith, Peggy Gragg, Arlene Gross, Bonnie Gudis, Cheryl Gutmacher, Judy Haley, Patti Keenan, Carol McGrath,

Ms. Singer, Ellen Smith, Joanna Southerland, Audrey Wallock, and those who requested anonymity.

Without their help, input, and encouragement, we could never have written this book.

PREFACE

This book is a collaboration among Sale, Woody, and Casey
Johnson, a family living with Type-I diabetes every day, and
writer-researcher Susan Kleinman. But because so much of
the information is based on Sale and Woody's experiences
and we wanted to capture what it's like to manage a child's
diabetes, we chose to write the first chapters in their first-
person voices, using their proper names only when necessary to avoid confusion.

Some of the other parents we interviewed requested anonymity. To respect their wishes, we have identified them
only as "a mother we spoke to," or "another mother we
interviewed," but have used the names of those parents who
gave us permission to do so.

Finally, and most importantly, while we have taken great
pains to ensure that all the information in this book is accurate, it is intended *only* for informational purposes, and
should never replace or override the advice of a competent
medical specialist. Diabetes is a complicated disease that
requires proper medical care, and the authors, publisher,
and contributors to this book cannot be held liable for the
consequences of any use or misuse of the information
herein.

CONTENTS

F O R E W O R D

Mary Tyler Moore
International Chairman,
Juvenile Diabetes Foundation International

I never talked about my diabetes until the Juvenile Diabetes Foundation started talking about a cure. From the time I was diagnosed in 1964, I worked almost as hard to keep my diabetes a secret as I did to keep it in control, fearing that if I told people I was diabetic they would look at me differently.

But, finally, I realized that I had to share my story — not just to help others, but also so that others could help *me,* with their encouragement, with their empathy, and with their optimism. When I was first introduced to the Juvenile Diabetes Foundation, I found myself swept up into an organization whose volunteer and professional staff were irresistible. Their confidence was exhilarating and their determination was clear: through research, they were going to cure diabetes.

Since then, in my role as International Chairman of JDF, I have met and worked with so many wonderful families, like the Johnsons, who are dedicating their lives to living with hope, and to turning those hopes into realities. But the Juvenile Diabetes Foundation — and *Managing Your Child's Diabetes* — are about more than just hoping for a cure. They're about making the days until that cure is found better for diabetics all over America . . . and all over the world.

In this book, you'll learn not only how to dream for the future, but how to cope with today, the way so many families of diabetics are doing. In these pages, a fourteen-year-old and her parents share their experiences with diabetes and their conviction that a cure for the disease will be found. They share medical information and coping strategies, parental advice, and a teenager's candor. And, in *Managing Your Child's Diabetes,* the authors share the optimism that has fueled their tireless work on behalf of diabetes research since Casey was diagnosed. That shared support and hopefulness are exactly what make *Managing Your Child's Diabetes* such a special and important book—and what make me wish this book had been available to me when I first was diagnosed.

The Johnsons' optimism is not just inspiring, it's contagious. I hope that as you read through these pages, their optimism gives you the strength to get through this very difficult time in your life, and the determination to fight with us against diabetes.

There *is* a cure for diabetes. If all of us—diabetics, parents, and friends—work together, I believe that we will find it.

INTRODUCTION

It's the stuff of TV melodrama: A seemingly healthy child goes for a routine checkup and the doctor discovers diabetes. But this isn't television, it's real life — *your* life — and the life of your precious child. There are no one-hour solutions, no miniseries miracles; just grief and anxiety and sometimes utter, hopeless despair. Why you? Why your child? How are you ever going to get through this?

Those are just some of the questions we asked ourselves when we discovered that our daughter Casey, who was then eight years old, has insulin-dependent diabetes. Even now, we remember clearly how we felt in those first few days after her diagnosis: we felt frightened, angry, and alone. Chances are, if you've picked up this book, you're feeling much the same way. Perhaps you've just learned of your child's illness. Or maybe you're having a rough time coping with the everyday challenges of raising a diabetic child.

No matter what your situation, no matter how isolated you may feel at this moment, you are not alone. In the six years since we discovered Casey's illness, we've learned an awful lot about diabetes, and about insulin, and about doctors' offices. But the most important thing we've learned is that we *are not* alone. We're in this not just with one another, but with the millions of other families dealing with diabetes. We may not all share hobbies, or time zones, or religious beliefs. We may not know each other personally. But what we share with all parents raising a diabetic child is the desire to keep our kids healthy, happy, and well-adjusted. What we'd like to share with *you* are many of the facts and strategies we've learned that make it easier to fulfill that desire.

By now, handling Casey's diabetes is second nature to us — and it's second nature to her, too. We may not love the fact that our daughter has diabetes, but because we love our daughter, we've had to accept her diabetes as part of our lives. We've tried, through our involvement in the Juvenile Diabetes Foundation, to make it not just a factor in our life, but a motivating factor. (There's nothing to get you moving like worrying about your child's health and her life!) As parents of a diabetic, we decided early on that we would do whatever we could to help in the search for a cure. We researched organizations devoted to helping diabetes patients, and for a while, we even thought of starting our own organization. But then we learned that there already was an organization working toward the only *real* remedy for diabetes: a permanent cure.

The Juvenile Diabetes Foundation does more, each year, to find that as-yet-elusive cure than any other organization. The Foundation's unique screening process allows JDF to find and fund research projects by the most brilliant minds working in the field today and, increasingly, in other fields that can shed light on the causes and cure for diabetes.

This is the time to find that cure, in this decade, in this golden age of science. We've read that there are more scientists alive today than in the history of humanity combined. Now, we *knew* there were more *lawyers* alive today than in all of history combined, but this fact about scientists boggled our minds. But it's true. Medical knowledge is expanding at a staggering pace today, and we're confident that one day soon, there will be a cure for diabetes.

In the meantime, we're determined to help Casey live as normally as possible. That isn't always easy, but it can be easier—and it has become easier for us, in the last six years—knowing that there are other parents out there (and experts, as well) who are willing to share their experiences, their knowledge, and their caring. That's why we wrote *Managing Your Child's Diabetes.* Knowing firsthand how overwhelming a child's diabetes can be, we wanted to share some of our own experiences and the experiences of other families, to let you know that you are not alone.

As important as moral support is, we know that sheer empathy won't help you find a specialist, or wade through medical forms, or coordinate your child's dietary schedule with her fifth-grade math teacher. So, drawing on some of the lessons we've learned through trial and error, as well as the advice of dozens of other parents, children, doctors, psychologists, teachers, and experts in various fields, we have attempted to offer an accessible, useable guide to managing your child's diabetes—organizationally, emotionally, and practically.

In the course of the interviews we conducted, we heard over and over again that there's no one right way to handle the challenge of a child's illness, but there are *better* ways— ways that can help minimize stress, maximize optimism, and keep your family as functional as possible.

We found that people were eager to share their stories with us—sad stories, triumphant stories, stories that make a point and drive it home. Some of the stories we tell in *Managing Your Child's Diabetes* were shared by everyone we spoke with, whether their child is six or sixteen: The first insulin shock is equally unnerving for babies and teenagers alike, and invariably leaves their parents a little bit strung out and a whole lot *wrung* out; watching a child you love go through rapid and unfamiliar body changes is scary for everyone.

Other insights and stories we heard were as unique as the special people who shared them with us. We heard about the problems that can occur when a vindictive ex-spouse cancels a child's medical insurance, and about the triumph a child feels when, because of his positive attitude, he is chosen to be a counselor in a summer camp for kids with diabetes. We heard sad stories and funny stories, instructive stories and stories that made us feel like we knew the people who told them, although we had never met.

Then we sat down to remember some stories of our own. The past six years have taught us a lot about ourselves and about each other, and have forced us to develop a lot of tricks and coping mechanisms we thought would be helpful to you.

Chief among these is: *listen* to your child. Raising a diabetic child — or any child, for that matter — is not a one-way street with textbook rules, but an ongoing process that has to change as your child and your situation do. Only your child can tell you how she's feeling today; only she can let you know if there's a problem with a teacher or classmate. That's why the first chapter of this book is told from Casey's point of view. We hope her account of what it's like to *be* a child with diabetes is helpful to you and your family as you work through the maze of emotions, practicalities, and challenges that are all an unspoken part of your child's diagnosis. We hope that as you read *Managing Your Child's Diabetes,* you become not only more aware of what goes into raising a child with diabetes, but more confident of your ability to do so, for when it comes to diabetes management, confidence is key.

So please believe us when we tell you that the facts that seem so confusing today will seem clear — and familiar — in no time. Believe us when we tell you that while the anxiety that set in when you first heard your child's diagnosis never disappears completely, it will keep shrinking until you wake up one morning and realize that you're living a far more normal life than you initially imagined you would. Please believe — as we do — that there is a cure for diabetes. If all of us work together on behalf of our children, we'll find that cure, together.

Managing Your Child's Diabetes

1

Casey's Story

To tell the truth, having diabetes hasn't turned out to be as horrible as I thought it would. In the beginning, I was just terrified.

I had gone to the doctor's office for some tests in the morning, and he told me to come back after school. That afternoon, my mother and I walked into his office and he said, "Call the house and ask someone to pack a bag and bring it over to the hospital." I didn't understand what was going on, or why, but everything was happening so fast that there wasn't even time to ask questions.

I checked into the hospital and the nurses started taking my blood, and talking about this sickness called diabetes. I had never heard of diabetes before, *plus* I was the kind of kid who'd faint at the sight of blood, so you can imagine how scared I was!

What I remember most about my stay in the hospital was that it seemed like the doctors kept me up all night explaining things. I know my parents think this was great and really helpful, but to me it just seemed like I couldn't get any sleep, and I was scared because I had no idea what was going on. It was only after I went home, when I had time to let my head clear a little bit that I started to understand. When you find out you have diabetes, you want people around you to cheer you up, but you also need to be left alone a little bit, to let all the new and scary information sink in.

Once I did understand what diabetes is, I started to feel sorry for myself. But now I know that even though that self-pity is normal, it keeps you from getting on with your life. So if you or your child just found out about diabetes, try not to feel sorry for yourself. (These days, when I *do* start feeling sorry for myself, I remind myself of the things I have that lots of other kids — even healthy kids — don't. I have a great family, and really terrific friends, and when I think about how lucky I am in other areas, then it reminds me not to feel sorry for myself.)

One of the things that helped get me out of my "funk" at the beginning was meeting a lot of people who had diabetes and were still leading very active lives. One was a fifteen-year-old girl who rides horses competitively. That got me really excited because it made me realize I could still do active things. If your child has diabetes, try and get him or her to meet other people who have the same hobbies and have continued them even with diabetes. This will help *your* child get excited, too!

The funny thing is, now that I'm used to my diabetes and know that I can still live a fairly normal life, I don't like to play with other diabetic kids. All they want to do — even if they're the nicest kids in the world who I'd be best friends with otherwise — is talk about diabetes. Once I had a friend with diabetes sleep over for the weekend, and all she wanted to do was talk about it, and it made me feel awful. I felt like "Why can't I just be a normal kid, who doesn't have to talk about being sick?" With my regular friends, we talk about the usual fourteen-year-old things, and that makes me feel like I'm the same as everyone else. Another time, I had a ski instructor who had diabetes. He was a great instructor, but he would stop me in the middle of a mountain and say, "Let's test our blood." It drove me nuts!

But when your child feels better talking about her diabetes, you need to respect that, too. You've got to listen to what your child is telling you about his or her feelings. The point is, even though diabetes is now a big part of your child's life, it doesn't really change who she is inside, and it doesn't mean that she is going to be exactly the same as other kids with diabetes. That's why I think the best way for parents to deal with their child's diabetes is to try to take their child's position, and imagine what she might be going through. Not what *you* would feel if you had diabetes, but what your child — with *her* personality — might feel like.

Also, remember that things aren't always going to be the same as they are when you first find out about diabetes. Pretty soon, you'll get used to having a kid with diabetes, but at the beginning, it's scary and a little bit weird for everyone.

When we went home from the hospital after a week, everyone treated me a little differently. There were a lot of people in the house, and they all stared at me when I came home. At the beginning, I was afraid that people would treat me differently for the rest of my life, and I really didn't want that.

Now, my family treats me pretty much the same as they treat my two sisters, but my teachers still treat me differently. For example, if I get a C on a test (which I try not to do!), they'll say "Good work," because they know I have a lot of other pressures because of diabetes. I like the encouragement, but I also know that because other people are willing to make allowances for my diabetes, it's up to me to keep my own standards high. It's up to me to know that getting a 'C' isn't such good work for me, no matter how nice the teachers are trying to be.

What's *hard* about having diabetes in school is that when I'm late for class or I skip gym, I wonder whether people think I'm using my diabetes as an excuse. But that's not the hardest part. For me, the worst part about having diabetes is when I'm having a great time with friends and I have to get up and leave to give myself a shot or test my blood. But when I let it go, I can have a mood swing, and that's even worse!

When your blood sugar gets too high, you have a mood swing, and when it gets too low, you can have a mood swing, too. When it gets low, you want to ignore the fact that you're having a low-sugar problem, so you talk a lot and you get really annoying and people get mad at you, so you blow up. If your blood sugar gets too high, you get incredibly hyper, and then you just blow up again.

Fortunately, I've had very few mood swings in school. I try so much harder to control myself there, because I know that if I keep blowing up, I won't have a lot of friends. At home, it's much more casual, and I'm more likely to just let a mood swing go without taking care of it. I don't know why I deny the reaction; it would be more logical to just go drink some juice and feel better, but I think that deep down I just don't want to accept the fact that I have diabetes, and the low-sugar feeling is a reminder that I'm different.

Another thing I hate dealing with is wearing my medical-alert bracelet, and I take it off as *soon* as I get home, because it drives me nuts. I know that if it was my choice, I would wear it, because I know it can really help me in an emergency. But because I *have* to wear it, it makes me not want to. That's reverse psychology for you!

That's the thing about diabetes: it feels so much better when you are in control of the situation yourself, and don't have to be told what to do all the time. For example, when I started giving myself my own shots a few years ago, it helped me to feel more grown up. I wasn't as dependent on my mother anymore, and that helped me feel more in control. At first, giving myself shots kind of grossed me out, but it also made me feel more in control — and my parents definitely understand that I like being in control, and they're really great about giving me some room to be more and more independent.

There are some other things you can do, too, to make things easier for your child with diabetes:

1. When you find out about the diabetes, don't fall apart in front of your kid. It's so hard for a kid to see her parents crying, especially if we feel like it's our fault. Of course, it's normal for you to be sad and scared if your child has diabetes (if you weren't, your child would think you didn't care!) but if you really go to pieces in front of your child, she'll feel like she's responsible for making you so upset, and she may even feel as if you're embarrassed about her diabetes. So try to save the really bad reactions for when you're not with her. (My parents would talk and cry after I was asleep.)

2. Don't embarrass your child in front of her friends or teachers or *your* friends and relatives. I hate it when my parents tell other people about my diabetes in front of me. I don't mind telling people myself, but when my parents do it while I'm standing there (like if they're giving instructions to a friend's parent before I go over) it makes me feel over-protected.

3. Try to find a good balance between ignoring your child and bugging her. When my mom bugs me about testing my

blood or taking my shot, I say "Leave me alone!" but then, when she does leave me alone, I wonder, "Doesn't she still love me?" Of course, I know she does, and I know my parents are trying to teach me to be independent and be in control.

I think that is the most important thing for you to know if your child has diabetes: Yes, she needs your support. And if she's young, she needs your help, too. But we kids with diabetes like to feel like we can take care of ourselves . . . like *we* can control our illness.

Every diabetic *can* do a lot to control her diabetes! I know that if I exercise and follow my doctor's instructions about food and shots, and if I check my blood-glucose levels when I'm supposed to and work hard to keep them in control, I can really make a big difference in my health — and in my life! Knowing that makes diabetes a lot less frightening.

So remember that things aren't always going to be as scary for you and your child as they are when you first hear about diabetes, and that believe it or not, a few good things can come out of diabetes. For example, I definitely got closer to my parents since I got diabetes, because I had to spend a lot of time with them for my shots. Even though I drive them nuts with my mood swings sometimes, we have really learned to trust each other and work together as a team, which a lot of families never experience.

Also, remember that things are getting better and better for diabetics: insulins are improving all the time, doctors are learning more about why people get diabetes and how to control it, and brilliant scientists, like my Uncle Alan, are working really hard to find a cure. When you get down in the dumps try and think about that. Try and remember that if you and your child work together to handle the diabetes, your life can be pretty normal . . . and just as exciting as everybody else's!

Now that I'm a teenager and more independent, I find that diabetes plays a much smaller part in my life. I have chosen to be less involved in fund-raising activities right now, and to spend more time with kids my own age who don't have diabetes but have lots of other things in common with me. It's great to know that supportive organizations like JDF are out there with help and activities if you want them, but I've really learned that what works best for me is trying to make diabetes as insignificant a part of my life as possible.

I think part of the reason I'm less focused on diabetes now is that taking care of myself gets easier all the time. The blood glucose checks and the shots are just something I do now, like waking up and brushing my teeth. I admit it—I don't always take care of myself as well as I should, and I'm not sure exactly why that is (except for the fact that you don't find a whole lot of 14 year olds anywhere doing just what they're supposed to!).

I guess it takes everyone a while to strike the right balance: you want to learn about diabetes and take care of yourself, but still feel like other kids and have a normal life. As I get older, I'm trying to find that balance. I'll probably make some mistakes along the way as I try out different ways of dealing with my diabetes—or *not* dealing with it, because lots of times all I want to do is ignore it! But the most important thing I've decided is that I have a right to try different ways of coping with diabetes and seeing what works best for me.

That's my wish for other kids with diabetes, too: Find out what's available, in terms of support systems and medical paraphernalia. But when it comes to making choices about how involved to get in organizations or whether a schedule your doctor wants to change you to is better than the one you're on now, THINK FOR YOURSELF, even if you're not old enough to make the ultimate decision yet. *You* are the one who has to live with your diabetes. And *you* have to find a way to make it interfere as little as possible with the things you ultimately want out of life.

Remember: the trick is to control your diabetes, and not let your diabetes control you!

2

Diagnosis and Hospitalization

Perhaps you had an idea, before your child's diagnosis, that something was wrong. Maybe you took her to the doctor because you were worried about her sudden weight loss. Maybe you called your pediatrician to find out why your nine-year-old was suddenly wetting her bed every night. Most of the parents we interviewed took their child to the doctor because of excessive thirst and urination. Maybe you even suspected diabetes. "I kept telling my pediatrician that Justin had diabetes and he thought I was crazy!" said one mother we interviewed. Or maybe, like us, you were taken completely by surprise.

In the spring of 1988, we were down in Florida on vacation. We stopped in to visit with Dr. Edward Saltzman, a friend of ours who is a pediatrician. He offered to look at our three daughters because they all had the chicken pox (what a vacation!). "Dr. Eddie" gave Daisy, Jaime, and Casey each a complete check-up, including urine and blood tests, and reported to us that we had three terrific, healthy kids . . . with chicken pox.

A few weeks later, we needed school forms filled out. We took all three girls to their pediatrician, Dr. Edward

Davies, in New York. When we left his office, the nurse said, "Congratulations! You have three healthy daughters!" But by the time we had made the ten-minute trip home, the nurse had called. She asked us to bring Casey back for a second urine test.

As Sale recalls, "I thought 'Oh, maybe she has a bladder infection or something.' So we took Casey's morning urine in the next day, and waited . . . until the waiter came over to me in the middle of a business lunch and told me I had an important phone call. It was Dr. Davies calling to tell me I had to bring Casey back to his office after school. When we got there, the doctor checked her urine again and then told us the bad news: He thought our daughter had diabetes."

We were stunned. Hadn't Casey just had her blood tested in Florida? Hadn't "Dr. Eddie" told us she was perfectly healthy? How could things change so quickly?

We immediately got on the phone to Sale's brothers; one, Dr. Alan Frey, holds a Ph.D. in molecular biology and the other, Dr. Jim Frey, is a neurologist. We figured that if anyone could explain to us what was going on, they could.

Jim told us that the urine-test results meant one of two things: kidney disease or diabetes — neither one of which is very good. Alan told us to redo the test, which we did. Like most parents who hear that their child might be ill, we liked the idea of another test. We hoped it would prove that there had been some terrible mistake, and that Casey was as healthy as every other little girl her age.

Thank goodness Dr. Saltzman's examination had been so thorough. He had tested her urine and found nothing unusual in the results. So we knew when it was diagnosed that Casey's diabetes had only begun very recently. As it turns out, the rapidity with which Casey was diagnosed worked in her favor. At the time we found her diabetes by accident, she'd been sick less than six weeks and her blood-sugar level was 364. Many children are only diagnosed when they've been ill long enough to start looking and feeling sick, and their blood sugar's way up even higher than Casey's. But because we hadn't recognized any signs of illness, Casey's diagnosis was even harder for us to believe. (The signs of course, were there: excess thirst and urination, no weight gain.)

But Dr. Davies said, "Look, we're just wasting time here. Casey needs to go to the hospital." Our hearts started pounding. Our heads started spinning. One day the doctors were telling us that we had wonderfully healthy kids, and the next, they're telling us our daughter has a life-threatening disease. If you've just been through this yourself, you know how very frightening and confusing the whole experience is. When the doctor told us that we didn't even have time to go home and throw some of Casey's belongings in a suitcase, we knew that this was very serious.

The few days that followed went by in a blur. On top of the stress of learning our child was diabetic, we had to cope with an encyclopedic mass of medical information. The doctors were speaking not just in medical terms, but in complicated biochemical jargon. That kind of jargon is all but impossible to comprehend when you're in shock, as we were. Friends would call and say, "So, what's going on?" and we didn't know how to answer. We weren't quite sure what was going on ourselves.

Looking back on it now, we know that our utter confusion was typical. Stress levels were at an absolute peak. The doctors were inundating us with information — information that would be complicated even in normal circumstances.

When your child has just been diagnosed, the information can seem even more confusing, because you just can't focus. You feel really helpless even though there are so many people helping you, and you're so worried that you're missing all the important information. That can make you even more nervous, which makes the whole thing worse.

Sale remembers it this way: "By the third day of Casey's hospital stay, we were getting really worried, because the doctors had been talking to us nonstop and we had understood very little of what they were telling us. So I called Paula Liguori, the nurse-educator who's part of our doctor's team and said, 'I don't understand any of this and somebody has to explain it to me in non-medical terms.' As soon as I had let out my frustrations, I started crying. And you know the lyrics of that old kids' song, 'It's all right to cry; crying gets the hurt out faster.' Well, it's true. I felt so much better after I'd really cried that I started to relax and understand what the medical staff was telling me."

So if your child's just been diagnosed and you're holding back the tears, let them flow. Crying will not only make you feel better by releasing the stress, but will also clear your head so that you can understand the complicated information you're receiving. Letting "the hurt out" can be very helpful when you're trying to let the information in.

Believe us, there will be *plenty* of information. In those first few days and weeks, you'll be swamped with facts, figures, and scientific data. You may find it hard to sort through it all and prioritize well enough to concentrate on what you need to learn first. In fact, many families — including ours — find, when they're getting ready to leave the hospital, that they're faced with the same panic that accompanied their trip home with a first newborn. There's no way to eliminate that nervousness entirely, but you can minimize it by making sure that you spend the bulk of your time in the hospital with your doctor or nurse-educator developing a basic management plan, with the following steps:

Recovery: Of course, you'll want to get your child as healthy as possible, as quickly as possible, so that you can bring her home from the hospital. To this end, the doctors will be experimenting with insulin levels that will bring glucose levels close to normal, and with a diet that works best with the way your child's body metabolizes food. The fine-tuning process will continue after you go home and throughout your child's life. But for now, the doctors will be working hard to get your child's glucose levels into an acceptable range.

Prevention: Your doctor or nurse-educator will spend time with you going over the signs of high and low blood sugar, and will teach you how to avoid these two risks. You'll learn how to monitor glucose levels, how to detect an impending reaction, and how to give your child her shots. (Naturally, your child's participation in all of these procedures will vary with her age.)

Make sure everyone who is responsible for your child's care learns the basics, as well. Right after Casey was discharged from the hospital, we had the nurse-educator, Paula Liguori, come and give a teaching lecture for the people at home and a few extended-family members. We all tested each other with shots and finger-sticking, and Paula explained to the babysitter and housekeeper about the exercise and the food, so that if we weren't there, Casey would still be in good hands.

If you can't set up a professional session at home, instruct the members of your household yourself. Your baby sitter and close relatives should all develop the skills and the confidence to oversee your child's diabetes-control routine if you are not available.

It's important for people around you to learn about diabetes not only for practical reasons (in case your child has an insulin reaction in your absence, for example), but so that they can become comfortable with your child and treat her as normally as possible.

Early intervention: Your doctor and diabetes educator will work with you to make sure you're clear about what to do if, even with all your preventive steps, there's a crisis. Do you know how to handle a glucose reaction? How to inject glucagon? How to reach your doctor in an emergency? Your doctor will go over all these things with you, and we'll review them in later chapters. Do not wait for a crisis to ask the doctor your questions. Ask them *now.*

Finally, you'll need to learn how to use the "tools of the trade" effectively. The doctors will send you home with a whole kit of syringes and glucose monitors, but they won't do you any good if you don't have the knowledge and confidence to use them. Few of us are comfortable with needles at first. But, ultimately, you and your child will become comfortable enough with the syringes to use them properly at home. How do you get to that comfort level? The same way you get to Carnegie Hall: practice, practice, practice!

We did a lot of practicing ourselves during those first few days in the hospital. We gave each other shots with saline solution to get the hang of the injections and to know what they felt like to Casey. We all took turns testing our blood until the procedure felt natural. "It took me a couple of days just to get the nerve up to prick my own finger," Sale remembers. "I would sit there and hold the lancet on my finger, waiting for the courage to stick myself." Casey herself has never had a problem with this test — and there's a lesson in that: Kids haven't had as much time as we adults have to develop a fear of doctors and needles, so they are often a lot more calm about shots and pinpricks than we are. Be careful not to get a calm child hepped up about a shot just because *you* find it frightening!

Our doctor and nurse-educator walked us through all the procedures. Led by Fredda Ginsberg-Fellner, M.D., who is still Casey's doctor, they stayed with us until 10:30 at night, every night, teaching us how to care for Casey.

Describing those first few days now, we realize that they had an Alice-in-Wonderland quality to them. We had tumbled into this strange new world of diabetes management, and we were spending so much of our time trying to adapt and find a happy ending.

Because you are experiencing so much that is new, you and your family members will probably react to what's happening in different ways. For example, we discovered, as we sat down and recalled the details of Casey's hospital stay for this book, that the same doctors who are forever enshrined in our hearts for helping Casey through her medical crisis are etched into *her* memory as "the guys who kept waking me up at night and bothering me."

As you cope with your own reactions to the diagnosis, your child is going through a series of feelings herself— feelings that may be hard for her to sort out, or even to understand fully. If your child is old enough to do so, encourage her to write her feelings down in a journal. This provides a much-needed steam valve.

Don't be surprised if your child seems to regress to a less mature level than she's been at for some time. Children in hospitals often become increasingly dependent on their parents. In fact, you may be surprised to find that *you* are suddenly more dependent on your own parents than you have been in a very long time. Sure, you're an adult, but the truth is that when trouble sets in most of us "want our mommies."

Remember that your child's reaction to his diagnosis will depend on his personality and his age. Casey was eight when she was diagnosed, which was old enough for her to understand what was going on and young enough to still be flexible about changing her lifestyle. Parents of infant diabetics have told us that the hardest thing about the diagnosis was dealing with a child too young to know what's going on, and parents of teenagers have complained that diabetes pits them against their children in a never-ending battle over shots and diet.

Of course, while you're coping with your child's reaction to the news that she has diabetes, you'll undoubtedly be experiencing a whole set of complex emotions yourself. We all go through the anger, the guilt, the confusion. We all go through the despair. Maybe you think you're the only parent to ever ask yourself what you did wrong to deserve this. The answer, of course, is nothing! Diabetes is an unpreventable disease, and nothing you did or didn't do caused it. Or perhaps you feel rotten because you think you're the only parent to ever feel angry at your child for getting sick, then guilty about your irrational anger. Well, think again.

"The guilt that we somehow gave our daughter this disease was so pervasive it was hard for us to concentrate on anything else," said one mother we interviewed. Another mother, who is still angry more than ten years after the diagnosis, wrote: "I can't believe those people who say diabetes improved their lives. Do they like worrying?"

But most parents ultimately get used to the worrying and overcome the common but irrational guilt. We can't stress strongly enough how important it is to try and retain your sense of optimism. Believe it or not, you'll soon adjust to your child's diabetes and you'll soon be able to laugh and smile again. In fact, there *are* families who feel that their child's diabetes has brought them closer or given them a finer appreciation of life. But at the beginning, *everyone* is thrown for a loop. Although every family and every situation are different, it's amazing how similar parents' reactions are when they learn their child has diabetes. According to experts at the National Information Center for Handicapped Children and Youth in Washington, D.C., there are many common reactions to the news that a child has a chronic disease.

First, there is denial. You hear the doctor's words, and you think, "She must be mistaken." You remember reading in the paper about hospital labs that mixed up patients' blood tests, about technicians who got lazy and didn't double-check results. You ask that the test be redone a second and third time. (In retrospect, we wonder how many re-tests we would have asked for if our doctor had not wisely and firmly told us to get Casey to the hospital.)

It can take days for the reality to set in, but ultimately you will come to realize, as we did, that the doctors *are* right. Your child really does have diabetes.

Then the anger sets in. We kept asking ourselves: Why is this happening to Casey? Why is this happening to us?

Lots of parents facing a new diagnosis feel angry at life, at the doctors, at God. You may even feel even angry at your child, though you know, rationally, that the diabetes isn't his fault. This anger, in turn, may provoke guilt. You know it's irrational to be angry at your child, but somehow you can't help it. Does that make you a horrible person? Of course not.

Perhaps you feel guilty, too, about "giving" your child diabetes, or about not identifying it earlier. In the beginning, it seems, every parent says, "I should have seen the signs sooner." But don't be too hard on yourself. Most people wouldn't recognize the symptoms of diabetes if they developed the disease themselves, let alone if they had to identify it in another. In fact, 50 percent of adult diabetes is untreated because its victims are completely unaware that they have the disease.

Before Casey was diagnosed, she was acting up a lot at the dinner table, often to the point where we'd have to ask her to leave the table and go to her room, because we didn't think it was fair that she was rude and disruptive to the rest of the family. This was before we knew she had diabetes. Once Casey was diagnosed, we realized that her outbursts may have been related to blood-sugar swings, and that she couldn't help her behavior. We felt tremendous guilt when we realized she had been sick and we were punishing her for it. We had only been doing what we thought was best. Luckily, this only went on for a few weeks, because Casey was diagnosed so quickly, but the guilt was still there.

Many parents feel guilty because they imagine that somehow they "gave" their child the disease. While diabetes is a genetically carried disease, it's not something we "give" our children, anymore than we "give" them Aunt Gloria's blond hair or the beautiful singing voice that no one else in the family shares. There is nothing you could have done or avoided during pregnancy to eliminate the disease, and no precautions you could have taken to prevent it from showing up.

Of course, none of these facts will keep you from feeling guilty. We went through enough of that same guilt ourselves to know that. Sometimes, parents' guilt leads to self-deprivation. But remember: Denying yourself the pleasures you enjoy won't make your child well. With all the additional stresses we parents of diabetics face, our family philosophy is to try and make every other aspect of our life as enjoyable as possible. An illness in the family can make everyone realize how precious life really is, and how foolish it is to waste any opportunity for joy.

After the initial guilt passes, after buckets of tears and days of agonizing self-torture, the reality starts to set in. Your child has diabetes. Even though diabetes is not, when monitored and controlled, an immediately life-threatening disease, every parent of a diabetic child feels terrified. How will we take care of our child? What happens if we give a shot incorrectly, or forget one altogether? Especially if your child is too young to assume any responsibility for diabetes control herself, you may feel overwhelmed by the fear that you'll have to be watching her every minute of her life for the next eighteen years. But we'll say it again, because we think it bears repeating: Things *will* get better. They will get easier much more quickly than you might imagine. Every diabetic's parent we spoke to went through the feelings you're experiencing, every psychologist we consulted acknowledged them, and every research study we read confirmed them. Your feelings of helplessness will subside quickly enough, but remember, while you're going through them, that you aren't alone. Having these feelings is all part of the mourning process.

Yes, mourning. For even when a child's life is not in immediate danger, it's natural to mourn the "loss" of our child's health, of her carefree youth, of our own freedom to pick up on a moment's notice and leave the kids with a next-door neighbor. "You are grieving the death of your child's perfect health," says Ellen Smith, whose daughter Debbie was diagnosed at age nine, "and you go through all the stages that you do when someone close to you dies."

"For a moment," says Penny Buschman, R.N., M.S., C.S., Assistant Professor at Columbia School of Nursing in New York City, "your child seems like a complete stranger." Furthermore, she notes, "Parents who learn that their child has diabetes aren't just reacting to the news that their child is sick today, but reacting to the fact that the child will have this condition all her life."

But luckily, *this* grief will change to relief when you realize that even with her diabetes, your child's life can be a long one, a happy one, and, thanks to advances in diabetes science, an increasingly healthy one.

To get through the initial tidal wave of feelings, don't deny them. Allow yourself to feel them. But try not to let them control you or make you act in extreme ways. According to Leonard Felder, Ph.D., author of "When a Loved One Is Ill," parents may react to a child's diagnosis in one (or a combination) of four self-destructive ways:

There's the "super-trooper," who insists she can get everything done herself. She (or he) often refuses help from well-meaning relatives, refuses to ask nurse-educators for assistance.

On the flip side, there are parents who act as if they can't be bothered with the details of caring for the chronically ill child. Obviously, if you're reading this book, you're not that parent, but maybe your spouse is. Has (s)he left all the details and responsibility to you?

Are you acting as a "boss" who starts telling everyone in

the family what to do and how to behave?

Or maybe, just maybe, you're fine on the sur,
carrying a time bomb inside, walking along as if
is fine — until the pressure is just too much to b

Obviously, none of these extremes is healthy — not for
you, not for your family, and ultimately not for your newly
diagnosed child. The balance we all strive for throughout life
is especially critical now. In dealing with your child's diagnosis — and with her diabetes, over time — resolve to do as
much as you can, but be willing to ask for help when you
need it. Let your feelings out, and admit, at least to yourself,
when the stresses of caring for a diabetic child are getting to
you. Talk your feelings over with your spouse (or with a
friend, if you're a single parent). Write them down, if that's
helpful to you. Lock yourself in the bathroom and scream, or
punch a pillow, or go to church. Do whatever you have to do
to deal with your child's diagnosis, so that you can keep a
clear head for all the information your doctor's about to give
you. For, as one mother we talked to pointed out, the time
right after your child is diagnosed can be stressful and confusing. "We muddled through our days in a haze," she told
us. "It was so hard to make decisions. Whether it was a
decision of what new car to buy or what to have for dinner,
every one was difficult. As we got into the routine, we were
able to think more clearly."

The more clearly you are able to think, the more clearly
you'll be able to explain to your child what's going on.
Nurse-practitioner Penny Buschman notes that during the
diagnosis and education process, many parents try to shield
their child from information. But as much as we all want to
protect our children from hearing about possible complications like blindness and amputations, it's important to help

your child understand as much about her body and her illness as she can. That way, she can become a more active participant in her care — and *that* can go a long way toward minimizing the risk of those complications!

What's more, letting your children know what's going on may actually help lessen their stress. Even young children will pick up on your tension whether you explain diabetes to them or not. If you *don't* clue them in about the problem, they're likely to imagine something far worse than the manageable reality of diabetes.

All parents inevitably learn that they can't shield their children from pain. You can't keep your son's first girlfriend from breaking up with him, and you can't keep the coach from benching your daughter for most of the soccer game. As parents of diabetics, we learn this hard lesson a little earlier.

If you're having trouble finding the right words to explain diabetes to your child, ask the nurse-educator for help; that's what she's there for. You might also find it helpful to read to your child a brochure written to explain diabetes. The Juvenile Diabetes Foundation (JDF) publishes booklets for newly diagnosed diabetic children, written in comforting, easy-to-read language that your child can refer to for a bit of demystification.

As difficult as it can be to explain the "tangibles" to your diabetic child, explaining the why's and the wherefore's can be even harder. Many parents told us that answering the simple question "why?" was the toughest task they'd ever faced as parents. Who among us knows how to answer when a child asks, "Why me?" (Who among us isn't wondering the exact same thing when we learn our child has diabetes?) Ultimately, Sale just tried to explain it to Casey the best way she could. She told her that everybody has their cross in life to bear and this is going to be ours, as a family. We reminded her of a school friend who has to have allergy shots once a week, and that her sister Jaime has to take allergy shots as well. Her friend and her sister have allergies to cats and dust, while she's allergic to sugar. To avoid a reaction they all take shots. It's important for children to understand that while their "cross" may be harder to bear than other people's, everybody has something to deal with that they'd probably rather *not* be dealing with.

For us — and for you — that "something" is Type-I diabetes. By now, perhaps, you've recovered from the bad news. But there's good news, too. While diabetes is one of the most dangerous diseases known to us, it is also one of the more manageable. There are lots of things you can do to cope better with your child's diabetes. There are things, too, that you can do to cope better with your diabetic child. That's what this book is all about. But before you turn the page and keep reading, take some time to come to grips with your feelings. Resolve that you and your child will manage her diabetes — and not the other way around.

And consider these helpful tips we've gathered from doctors and psychologists and diabetics' families across the country:

• Remember that your child's diabetes requires *your* strength. Stay healthy, sleep well, and get exercise.
• Develop an expertise in diabetes. Your knowledge will be reassuring to your child, and will also allow your family to become less dependent on doctors for simple information. Appendix A of this book has a listing of information sources, and many children's hospitals have resource libraries. These libraries are not only a great place to pick

up literature about diabetes, but often a good place to find other parents who know what you're going through.

• Buy your child a medical-alert bracelet saying she has insulin-dependent diabetes. Most kids hate to wear them (just ask Casey!) but we can't stress enough how important proper identification is. It could actually save your child's life if she has a diabetic crisis when she's not around anyone who knows her.

• Get support. Become active in the Juvenile Diabetes Foundation (JDF), the American Diabetes Association (ADA), or both, and draw on the knowledge and experience of other families that have been through what you're going through now. Some JDF chapters (including the one in West Houston) are organizing programs in which diabetic children and their families visit newly diagnosed diabetics in the hospital to offer them the encouragement they need right from the start.

• If there are no support groups in your area, think about starting one yourself. Ask your doctor for the names and numbers of other families dealing with diabetes. Or, if you're in a small town without a large enough diabetic population to form a group, ask your pediatrician if she has any other patients with chronic illnesses. They may having coping strategies that will help you adjust to your child's diabetes.

• Talk about your feelings, but don't let them stop you from moving forward. "Don't let your child feel sorry for himself for too long," says Mrs. Singer, the mother of a seven-year-old boy. "Treat his diabetes as a condition, not a disease, so he doesn't think of himself as 'sickly.' "

• Think positively. Focus on ways of *preventing* complications, not on the complications themselves. Think about everything scientists are doing to find a cure for diabetes, and do the best you can, each day, in the meantime. "I wish I had relaxed more and not looked so far ahead to dwell on complications," said one mother, looking back. "Try to take your child's diabetes one day at a time."

• Get involved! "Participating in fund-raising activities is the best way to feel as if you're making a difference and empowering yourself," says Judy Haley, a JDF member who has two diabetic children. "Getting involved will give you a healthy outlet for the anger you might feel— it will help you turn that anger into action."

• When you are feeling angry, remember that the enemy is not your diabetic child, but diabetes itself, and that armies of researchers are on your side in fighting and trying to cure this disease. Don't let diabetes pit you and your child against each other in a battle of wills over shots and diet. Remember that until a cure is found, it's us and our kids *together* against diabetes.

3

Doctors and Hospitals

When our doctor made Casey's initial diagnosis and told us to get her to the hospital immediately, he suggested Mt. Sinai here in Manhattan, because there were endocrinologists who specialize in diabetes on call twenty-four hours a day. There were also construction workers on call twenty-four hours a day, since the hospital was in the middle of renovation. But we felt that the round-the-clock care Casey could get in the hospital and the quality of care she would receive after being discharged were worth putting up with the banging and the boarded-up windows. Mt. Sinai's Chief of Pediatric Endocrinology, Dr. Fredda Ginsberg-Fellner, became our diabetes specialist, and we've been very pleased with the way she and her team have cared for Casey ever since.

When we stop and think about it now, we realize how lucky we were to live in a city with more than one fine hospital to choose from and to have hooked up immediately with a doctor we trusted and felt comfortable with. We hope you'll be as lucky. But we also hope you won't leave finding your child's specialist *entirely* to luck. Finding the best doctor is so important not only because of the profound difference good blood-sugar control can make in your child's long-term health, but also from an emotional standpoint. As Shirley Swope, a parent advocate with the PEAK Parent Center in Colorado Springs, explains, "You have to put so much trust in this person who's sitting there telling you awful things about your child's body. When you have to give someone so much power over your life, it gets really scary. Initially, a child's illness is so overwhelming, you need someone who will guide you."

Guidance and kindness go a long way, but they must be accompanied by rock-solid expertise in diabetes. Lots of doctors say, "Oh yes, I know about diabetes," but staying current on what's going on in diabetes research and care is a full-time job. Indeed, diabetology is a field in which there's constant change, because of what researchers are discovering. Unless your doctor specializes in diabetes and attends all the conventions and the medical meetings, she's not going to be up on the latest developments in research and treatment.

Your pediatrician may have experience treating other diabetic children, but a specialist has treated hundreds or thousands of children with the disease, and can devote 100 percent of her time to increasing her knowledge of diabetes and 100 percent of her office budget toward whatever equipment and materials will help keep her office state-of-the-art.

Of course, not every family lives as close to a major diabetes treatment center as we do in New York City. You may be hours away from the nearest specialty center. But even if you have to make a big trip to a specialist, it's worth doing so a couple of times a year, especially at the beginning. As Barbara Davis says of the Center she founded in Denver in 1980, "It's a mecca of knowledge and support. A general physician will give you bits and pieces of advice as you need them, but at the Barbara Davis Center, children are taught everything they need to know: the shots, the nutrition, the motions. We are a research facility, and we're a facility where a diabetic child has someone to call 24 hours a day for advice or information or just to have a friend to talk to. As a result, children come here from around the world. We teach them how to live healthy lives with diabetes." (See Appendix C for a listing of diabetes-education and treatment centers accredited by the American Diabetes Association.)

Working closely with a specialist who can teach you the most up-to-date ways of controlling your child's diabetes, you will soon become something of an expert yourself. That, too, will help you ensure that your child is receiving the best care, not just during her office visits but every day, in every way.

Most families find their diabetes specialist through their regular pediatrician, and most of the parents we spoke with were perfectly content with the doctors they met this way. But we did hear a few complaints:

A mother in Chicago told us that "Unfortunately, at the time our daughter was diagnosed there was one doctor in the area that we all went to. He was very dogmatic and difficult to talk with. It seems that even doctors with excellent reputations resist questions and are very matter-of-fact and uninvolved."

"When doctors talk about complications," complained another parent, "they'll say things like 'But don't worry, only 10 percent of patients develop this problem.' They don't realize that is no reassurance at all for a parent whose child has a disease that affects only one in hundreds of Americans."

Another parent complained about doctors who treat you like "Case #12345-A, instead of the Jones family," and indeed, this coldness seems to be the most common complaint families have against their doctors.

It's important that you feel both you and your child can communicate with your diabetes specialist. Studies conducted at the Fox Chase Center in Philadelphia revealed that patients who were involved in their own care and were not afraid to ask questions felt more in control of their illnesses than those who followed their doctor's instructions blindly without dialogue. If you and/or your child can't talk freely with the physician, shop around for somebody else.

Yes, *shop.* Remember that with a doctor, as with every other service provider, you are the customer. "Just naming yourself a health-care consumer rather than a patient will give you a different orientation of who you are and what you should expect," Edward Krupat, Ph.D., director of the health-psychology program at the Massachusetts College of Pharmacy and Allied Health Science in Boston, was quoted as saying, in *SELF* magazine.

Many adults are more careful choosing their hairdressers or an auto mechanic than they are choosing their physician, but the choice of your child's diabetes-care specialist will affect not only her health but also the way she adapts to her diabetes and copes with it as she matures. So if you aren't pleased with the first doctor you're referred to, ask your pediatrician for other recommendations.

If your pediatrician does recommend a specific doctor, ask her *why* Dr. So-and-so? Often recommendations are based as much on friendship as on anything else. Remember that while your pediatrician's med-school buddy may have been a terrific study partner forty years ago, this doesn't guarantee her current level of expertise. Make sure the doctor who is doing the recommending has seen the specialist "in action" recently.

Another good way to find out about specialists is to ask the nurses in the hospital about different doctors. They'll know who has good reputations and who interacts well with patients, and will be less bound by the fraternal gag-order that sometimes keeps doctors from badmouthing one another even when bad press is called for.

If you want additional recommendations, ask other parents of diabetic children. If you have attended a support group, ask parents for the names of doctors they've been pleased with—and ask them *why* they're pleased. After all, if what they love about the doctor is that she can get them in and out of the office in fifteen minutes, you may not be comfortable if you like to know you can take your time. If they like a doctor because she's up on the latest biofeedback techniques, she may not be the choice for you, if you have a bias against unconventional medicine. Similarly, if you know another parent is much more neurotic than you, bear in mind that this may color her judgment about the doctor. You may feel differently about a doctor, too, if *you* are more high-strung than the parents making the recommendation.

Know thyself. And put that knowledge to work for you when you're hunting for a doctor. Even among great physicians, no one doctor is right for every patient or every family, so in addition to looking for a doctor with great qualifications, try to find one with a personal style you're comfortable with. For example, some doctors are uncomfortable with parents—or even kids—crying in their offices. If you're the "four-hankies-per-visit" type, this is not a doctor for you. Some doctors like to crack a lot of jokes. Will this put you at ease or make you feel the doctor's not taking your questions seriously enough?

Once you've gotten a list of specialists, set up appointments to meet with a few of them. You will have to pay for initial appointments even if you don't plan to use the doctor again, but it's money well spent if you're having a tough time finding a doctor you're pleased with. What should you be looking for? As we mentioned above, no one doctor is right for every patient or every family, but generally a good doctor is one who continually updates her practice and is a good medical detective. A good doctor also encourages the patient's independent thought and decision-making. The last thing you want is a practitioner who's going to manipulate you into believing that you can't make a simple decision about your child without her advice. Every parent we spoke to stressed that "You know your child better than any doctor." A good doctor respects your innate knowledge of your child, and applies it to her professional analysis of your child's medical situation.

Ultimately, finding the perfect doctor/patient fit involves a lot of intangibles and personality issues, but there are some concrete things you can look for when doctor shopping. For starters, take a look at the office walls—but don't be guided by the academic wallpaper alone. Remember: *Someone* has to graduate at the bottom of the class at Harvard Medical School, and there are plenty of "stars" from fine state medical colleges. Start by inquiring where your doctor did her residency and any fellowships. Is she board certified in pediatric endocrinology? You can call 1-800-776 CERT to confirm if a doctor is board certified.

Find out where the doctor has admitting privileges, too. If you have to rush your child to an emergency room in the middle of the night, will she be in a top-flight hospital? Are there specialists on call at the hospital twenty-four hours a day? Find out if your doctor will be in charge of your child's case any time she's admitted to the hospital. If not, why? Who will be? Ask to meet him or her.

If the doctor admits at more than one hospital, ask how she picks which of the hospitals you'll go to. Sometimes doctors have to fill quotas at each of their hospitals to retain their admitting privileges. That can make it difficult for them to make completely objective admitting decisions. Find out whether you can choose which of your doctor's hospitals your child will go to. Even among excellent hospitals, there are differences. At a teaching hospital, for example, your child will be exposed to medical students, and there can be as many as five extra sets of eyes gawking at her while she's treated. If this bothers her or you, you have the right to request that students, interns — or anyone other than your own physician — leave the room at any time. The extra eyes are not a bad price to pay, though, for the advantages major medical centers offer. They are often research centers; university-affiliated hospitals usually offer absolutely the latest in care.

Another thing to keep in mind when evaluating a doctor is her age. If you're looking to establish a long-term relationship with a physician so that she can see your child into adolescence and adulthood, you probably shouldn't start seeing a doctor who's six months away from retirement. On the other hand, someone who's still waving her med school diploma to dry the ink probably isn't your best bet, either.

Selecting a physician is one area in which it's acceptable (advisable, even) to be a snob. Don't hesitate to inquire how the doctor has been recognized for excellence. Is she a fellow

in the American Academy of Pediatrics subsection on endocrinology? Is she a member of the Lawson Wilkins Pediatric
Endocrine Society and the Council on Diabetes and Youth
of the American Diabetes Association, or otherwise affiliated
or recognized as being especially qualified to deal with your
diabetic child? Does she hold other academic or teaching
honors? Is she widely quoted in the press? Beware: That
isn't always a guarantee of excellence. If you see a doctor
quoted in the press or interviewed on TV, it means one of
two things: Either she is truly an expert in the field, *or* she
has made a career out of being a media doctor and cares
more about the person on the other side of a camera than the
one on the other side of a stethoscope.

A famous doctor does you no good if you can't speak to
her on the phone until after her six-month media tour or if
you only get to see her right-out-of-school associate. In the
first year or two that your child has diabetes, you'll want
frequent contact with your specialist (even if it's only by
phone between quarterly or semiannual checkups), so it's
important that your doctor be accessible. Find out what the
arrangements would be if your doctor isn't available. If there
are other doctors in the practice, be sure to meet with all of
them at least once in a non-emergency situation. If you're a
member of an HMO or are thinking of joining one, be sure
to meet with the doctors who would be treating you, and
make sure they are specialists. Many HMO services are well
equipped to deal with routine care but less stellar when it
comes to handling chronic or serious illnesses. If your HMO
does not have a specialist, you might want to see if you can
change plans.

Whether you're dealing with a solo doctor, a group practice, a clinic, or HMO setup, find out whom to call in an

emergency. "Make sure the doctor will give you his home number!" urges one of the mothers we interviewed. "You've got to know where to reach him in case of an emergency — at any time." Since you never know when your child is going to have a diabetic crisis, you'll want a physician who is accessible when you and your child need her. Besides a home phone number, make sure you ask the physician for her beeper number, too.

In addition to asking these basic questions, ask the doctor a few less obvious questions, as well. The experts at Colorado Springs' PEAK suggest that you cover the following points with any prospective physicians:

1. Ask the doctor how she feels about giving bad news. Does she think information should be withheld from parents?

2. What is the turnover rate of the office staff? If nurses and receptionists quit every three days, the doctor probably isn't that easy to get along with.

3. How flexible is the office about billing and payments? Diabetes can be an incredibly expensive disease, and if you're in tight or variable financial circumstances, it's important to know that the doctor will cut you a bit of slack in emergencies.

Sometimes, parents are afraid that asking "too many questions" will be misinterpreted as lack of confidence in their physician, or that if they question anything the doctors are doing, they'll seem ungrateful for the care they're getting. Many parents (of diabetics and nondiabetics alike) are secretly afraid that if they make the doctors angry, their children won't get the most compassionate care. Remember that it's not only your right but your obligation to your child to ask your doctor questions. If a physician discourages you from doing so, you can leave her office through the same door you walked in.

When you do ask your questions, don't just listen for the doctor's verbal answers. Watch how the physician interacts with your child and with you. Does she make eye contact? Does she seem distracted? Will she admit when she's wrong? Will she talk to you on a level that communicates that while you may not know all the words, you have the intelligence to comprehend the concepts? Will she take enough time to answer your questions? No doctor knows all the answers immediately; don't trust anyone who pretends to.

For further information on the doctors you are considering, you can contact the Public Citizen Health Research Group, 2000 P Street, NW, Suite 700, Washington, DC 20036. Its publication lists physicians across the United States who have been disciplined by state licensing boards. The Center for Medical Consumers, 237 Thompson Street, New York, NY 10012, publishes a newsletter, called *Health Facts,* that deals with ways consumers can get information on their doctors and hospitals.

Once you've chosen a diabetes specialist, she will probably help you put together your child's diabetes-management team. In addition to Dr. Ginsberg-Fellner and her associates, Drs. Robert McEvoy, Fenella Greig, and Signe Larsen, we spent a lot of time right after Casey's diagnosis with Paula Liguori, a certified diabetes nurse-educator. Paula was the one who taught us how to give Casey her insulin shots and how to test her blood. She was the one who sat down and talked to us in language that we could understand even after long stressful days in the hospital. Even now, we find it helpful to talk to her occasionally for advice on handling growing-up issues related to Casey's diabetes.

A certified diabetes educator (CDE) could be a nurse, dietician, pharmacist, or psychologist who has been specially trained and licensed to teach diabetics how to control their condition and care for themselves. Their licensing test includes medical information, and their practical training schools them in understanding what it's like to live with diabetes. There are more than 4,500 CDEs in the United States; write the American Association of Diabetes Educators at 500 North Michigan Avenue, Chicago, IL 60611, for a listing of those in your area if your doctor doesn't work closely with one.

Your child's diabetes-care team may also include a dietician or nutritionist who will help you plan an eating program, teach your child how to stick to it, and motivate her from time to time when her resolve to eat healthfully weakens. You'll probably call upon other specialists, including podiatrists, ophthalmologists, and psychological counselors, from time to time, as needed.

Because diabetes care is so multifaceted, and because there are often several specialists involved in your child's care, it is important for you (and your child, if she's old enough) to take charge of coordinating efforts among all the specialists. "Make sure that all the doctors on the team are consistent with philosophies, understanding, and instructions toward the parents," urges a mother active in JDF. "This makes it a lot easier for you to follow their instructions."

While all this conducting may sound a bit complicated and expensive, it actually simplifies life at no extra cost other than the few cents it might cost to make photocopies of your child's medical records for one doctor to send to the others.

Ideally, your pediatrician will be a good conductor, coordinating activities and reports from *all* your specialists, but ultimately it's up to you to request that all of the doctors keep your pediatrician apprised of your child's progress. If you shut your pediatrician out of your child's medical affairs, or start going to your specialist rather than the general children's doctor for routine checkups, you may find yourself in a situation where you need the pediatrician in an emergency and have to waste crucial time catching her up on the last two years of your child's medical history.

Sometimes, doctors are reluctant to copy their office records for other physicians, but your child's medical charts are yours *by law.* Ask for duplicates of everything. That way, you can photocopy your child's medical charts at a local copy shop whenever you want. Make sure your specialist has copies of your child's general medical records and that your pediatrician is kept up-to-date on what your endocrinologist observes.

In *A Parent's Guide to Asthma* (Doubleday, 1988) author Nancy Sander printed a parent's open letter to her specialist; her words are as relevant to the diabetic child's parents as to parents of an asthmatic: "As I see it," she wrote, "you and I are about to become a team. Our goal is to make this child as healthy as possible. You'll be the coach who sends in the plays from the sidelines, and I'll be the quarterback who sees that the plays are executed properly."

Experts at PEAK in Colorado offer several tips for making this "quarterbacking" easier:

First, everyone must accept the different roles of the various team members, and the inevitable differences of opinion about the child's needs. These differences are valuable, and should be a positive catalyst to help all the "experts" in the child's life create the individualized program that he or she really needs.

Second, people must be honest and share what they are thinking directly with each other. Parents must tell professionals their thoughts; professionals shouldn't have to presume or guess what parents are thinking.

Professionals have an obligation to be honest with parents. Protecting parents from difficult information is not an act of partnership. "In fact," say PEAK's experts, "if bad news is shared with parents in advance, they can come to a meeting best prepared to be effective, informed decision-makers in a business-like setting."

Sometimes, speaking up honestly is difficult for parents who are afraid of alienating the professionals their child depends on. However, not speaking up will only result in more stress and frustration in the long run.

For example, many parents told us that sometimes, it seems like their doctor is distracted while talking to them — opening her mail, going through her phone messages. There's no reason you can't express your annoyance at this. You don't have to rant and rave (that rarely accomplishes *anything!*). Just politely say: "I understand that you're very busy, but its important to me to feel that you're concentrating on what I'm saying." If the problem persists to the point that you start worrying whether the doctor *is* actually hearing what you say, you might want to switch to a more attentive and caring physician. You can usually avoid that kind of mid-stream horse-changing, though, if you work hard at developing positive communications skills — and that means sharpening your listening skills as well as your ability to articulate your questions. Humorist Fran Lebowitz says that the opposite of talking isn't listening — it's waiting to talk. Be sure you're attentive to your doctor's answers to your question, and not just waiting to ask the next one while she talks.

Communicating with your doctor shouldn't start and end at her office door. With a little advance preparation on your part, you can get more out of your routine visits and communicate better with your specialist in a crisis. Here are some thoughts we've gathered from other parents:

• Many of us are intimidated by doctors. Some adults even experience physical symptoms, like nausea or a rise in blood pressure, the minute they step into a doctor's office. This condition (called "white-coat hypertension") can often be minimized if you simply acknowledge it verbally.

• If you notice a problem, keep a journal of when it happens. Is your child always moody right before lunch time? Does she have a lot of low-blood-sugar episodes during exam week? Let your doctor know not just what's happening, but when. If you can correlate problems with their times or triggers, your doctor can be more helpful in finding solutions.

• Come to your doctor's appointment with a list of questions, and bring a pencil and paper for note-taking. Better yet, take a tape recorder. Unless you're a steno expert, taking notes can take your mind off what the doctor is really saying. Ask your doctor for permission to record her, and, if she doesn't mind, tape your conversation so that you can go over the specifics at home, and just write down the key points.

• Also, go with a clear objective: What is it you want to get out of the appointment?

• If your doctor is speaking too fast or using too much jargon, stop her now and then and ask "How do you spell that?" This trick not only helps you remember some of the more difficult words, but gently reminds the doctor that all of these terms are very new and unfamiliar to you. "The problem," says parent-advisor Shirley Swope, "is that doctors know the issues so well, they forget they're talking to someone who isn't as familiar with the terminology as they are. Sometimes, you just have to look at them and say, 'Excuse me, could you use sixth-grade vocabulary, please?' "

• Before you leave the doctor's office, ask yourself, "Has everything been explained to me clearly enough so that I can implement it at home?" Put your pride aside if you feel silly asking the doctor to repeat herself for a third or fourth time. Don't forget: This information has direct bearing on your child's health and well-being!

• After any meeting in which you've been asked to digest a lot of information, make a date to call the doctor in a few days to go over any points you don't understand. Sometimes, things make complete sense when you're sitting in the doctor's office, and then when you go home and look at your notes, it's all gibberish.

• Even today, most mothers are far more involved in the day-to-day aspects of their child's care than fathers are. *Whichever* parent goes to the doctor with your child, it's important to relay information to the other parent, to avoid freezing him or her out (and so that you can take advantage of the intelligent insights spouses are always coming up with when you least expect it!) Make sure to share information with your spouse and your babysitter (and your child herself, if she missed some of the information) as soon as possible after you talk to the doctor. This way the information will be freshest in your mind and any changes in care can be implemented immediately.

• To keep all the information you gather well organized, buy yourself a three ring binder and use it to store notes taken during visits along with copies of your child's medical records. Having an easy reference system readily available gives you one less point of stress to contend with before and after doctor's visits.

• Remember that no matter how responsive a doctor is to your needs, she won't know what those needs *are* unless you keep in touch. Call your specialist when your child's lifestyle has changed, when other kids in the house have a virus she might catch, or when you have any questions you'd like answered.

In addition to making the doctor visits as stress-free on yourself as you can, there are things you can do to make them less aggravating for your child.

• Before going to the doctor's office, explain to your child honestly what will be done. Don't do this too far in advance, though; a frightened child will experience that unpleasant medical procedure thousands of times in his mind before it actually occurs. Try to minimize the time your child has to dread the procedure.

• If you lie and tell your child an upcoming shot or test won't hurt, and it does, you lose the child's trust. Try to be honest without being frightening. If you have made decisions about honesty with your child, share them with your doctor, so that she can act consistently.

• Never, ever talk to the doctor about your child as if she isn't in the room. Teach your child, instead, to be as involved in her own care as she can from an early age. Encourage your child to be an advocate for herself, and to attend meetings with doctors even when they don't include examinations, so she gets used to dealing with physicians and working with them.

• After your child has endured a shot or an uncomfortable testing procedure, don't say, "That wasn't so bad, was it?"

Most of the time, it *was* pretty bad. Instead, say, "I know that was uncomfortable, but it's over now, and we can go home."

Over the years, your doctor will see you through numerous highs and lows—in blood-sugar level and emotions. And as your child and the science of diabetes management change, so will your doctor's advice. Throughout all the changes, try to retain your objectivity about the doctor and her suggestions, and to evaluate medical advice in terms of what you know about your child in your mind and what you sense about her in your gut.

Never be afraid to get a second opinion; it's not an insult to your doctor, as long as you don't phrase it as such. Just tell your doctor that as much as you trust her judgment you want to make your decisions with as well-rounded a view of the situation as possible. Doctors are used to this. Indeed, most professionals—and many insurance companies—expect you to get a second opinion before consenting to surgery or other major treatments. When you do get a second opinion, get one from a doctor at a separate hospital. Imagine the discomfort of working with someone who knows you're second-guessing him, and you'll understand why many doctors are reluctant to give anything but rave reviews to the colleagues they work with every day.

A second opinion may be especially valuable if you're evaluating a new or experimental method of diabetes control. Before starting your child on a new strategy or experimental approach, investigate the program: Who's running it? What has their success been with other experimental treatments? Talk with parents whose children are in the program, and with others whose children have discontinued it and find out why.

Then check whether your health-insurance policy covers

the program or physician. While this factor may not make your ultimate decision for you, it might play a part when you're deciding between two avenues of care.

Unfortunately, many insurers will pay for crisis care but not for preventive medicine. But waiting for a crisis to visit your doctor is not only penny-wise and pound-foolish, but risky to your child's life, as well.

No health-insurance policy will cover all of the expenses associated with diabetes care. The good news is, if your unreimbursed medical expenses exceed 7.5 percent of your adjusted gross income, many of them *are* tax deductible. So while you don't get all the money back, you pay less *in* at tax time.

According to Bernard Kleinman, C.P.A., A.P.F.S, the following diabetes-related expenses are tax deductible:

• Doctors' fees
• Fees for hospital services, including therapy, nursing services, ambulance times, and lab tests
• Payment for hospital room
• Prescription medications and insulin, but *not* medicines sold over the counter (like cold medicines, aspirin, etc.)
• The cost of transportation for visits to the doctor and hospital, including taxi and plane fare
• Your medical-insurance premiums
• Equipment, including syringes, glucose monitors, and ketone-test strips

On the other hand, extra babysitting help, your meals when visiting your child in the hospital, and social activities recommended by your physician (like camp) are *not* tax deductible. These are just guidelines; speak to your own accountant before making any claims on your tax return and keep careful records of your expenses. You can save a lot of money over time in tax deductions.

You can also save money by comparison-shopping for diabetes equipment; see Appendix B for the names and phone numbers of some supply houses that sell diabetic products at a discount.

No matter how tight money gets, try not to cut corners when it comes to frequent checkups. Besides being better for your child's health, frequent checkups lower the chances of a serious diabetic crisis that might require a trying (and very expensive) hospital stay.

Luckily, we haven't had to hospitalize Casey since her diagnosis, and many diabetic children can avoid having blood sugars so low or so high that they need to be checked back into the hospital—but it's always a good idea to have a worst-case-scenario game plan.

If you *do* have to hospitalize your child again for her diabetes or for any other reason, the following tips will make the experience easier on you and your child. (If you're reading this during your child's initial hospitalization, the following tips may be helpful today, too.)

• Find out if your doctor will be making regular visits to the hospital. How often? At what time? If it's possible, try and coordinate your doctor's visit with times both you and your spouse can be there. There is so much information to assimilate at first that the more competent pairs of ears you can get listening to it the better.

• If your hospital has a patients' representative, ask to meet her as soon as possible after admission. Find out when and where you can reach her if you have any questions about making the hospital stay easier, or any problems with doctors, nurses, or bureaucrats in the hospital system.

• Don't take any valuables to the hospital, as they have a way of disappearing. If your child wants her security blanket or a special doll, mark it with your child's name and ask the nurses and attendants to keep track of it to the best of their abilities.

• Bring pictures of other family members. Separation can be tough on young kids, and having pictures of siblings and pets can make it a bit easier.

• Be aware that not everyone called "doctor" in a hospital really is. In many medical places, the med students (including those who have been working on the wards for a day and a half) are called "doctor." Assume nothing.

• Most hospitals will let a parent stay overnight. Unless your child explicitly tells you otherwise, she probably wants you to stay; most kids do. In an article in the *American Journal of Public Health,* 1978, Barbara M. Kursch, M.D., wrote: "Parents must not only be allowed to visit, live in, or participate, they must be encouraged, supported, and educated to be the greatest possible help to the hospitalized child."

• If you or your child feel uncomfortable about the hordes of medical students or residents gawking at her during your doctor's visits, you may ask them to leave the room. Article 5 of the Patients Bill of Rights issued by the American Hospital Association states that "the patient has the right to every consideration of his privacy concerning his own medical-care program. Case discussion, consultation, examination, and treatment are confidential and should be conducted discreetly. Those not directly involved in his care must have the permission of the patient to be present." (Remember, though, that no one is born a doctor; the students in the room are there because they need to learn how to care for children like yours. So if you can tolerate their presence, at least part of the time, try to do so.)

If your child is admitted to the hospital for a non-diabetes-related cause (appendectomy, for example, or a broken bone) you must be especially careful that her diabetes-control regimen isn't disrupted.

A mother in Illinois told us, "I find it surprising that many emergency personnel don't know the basics about Type-I diabetes. We are frequently asked, 'Does your child take insulin?' and are shocked that the doctors and nurses aren't aware that almost *all* young diabetics are insulin-dependent."

Another mother told us, "When my daughter was in the hospital for knee surgery, we were amazed to see how many trained professionals don't know how to care for a diabetic. They tried to give her glucose instead of plain saline in her intravenous." If your child is having surgery, a diabetologist *must* be on hand to monitor her blood while she's under the anesthesia.

In addition to keeping an eye on the non-diabetes-expert doctors who may be caring for your child during a hospital stay, be sure to determine who is in charge of your child's food. If you are given a menu to select from, go over it with a diabetes-knowledgeable staff member. Don't assume that a regular floor nurse knows enough about your child's special diet. That's unfair to both her and your child.

If you keep your eyes open and your wits about you, you should be able to navigate the medical maze without too many problems. Most of the doctors we've come across are caring, competent practitioners who truly want to help children with diabetes live longer, healthier lives. If you shop carefully for your doctor and remain an active participant in your child's medical care until she's old enough to oversee it herself, you'll probably find that you can rely on your doctor to make sound decisions that work well for your child.

To educate yourself a bit better about some of the medical factors your doctor is likely to discuss with you, read the next two chapters on what diabetes is and how you can control it. If you'd rather skip to the other chapters first, be sure to review the medical information soon. Becoming diabetes-literate is one of the most important things you can do to make managing your child's diabetes easier.

4

What Is Diabetes?

It's hard to remember a time when we *didn't* know about diabetes, but like most parents, we were completely naïve about it when Casey was first diagnosed. Sure, we knew it was a serious disease, but we knew nothing about ways we could minimize its seriousness by helping her lessen the risk of long-term complications. We had no idea how she got diabetes, or whether it was possible to get rid of it. We wondered how many other kids had diabetes, and whether our two younger daughters would develop diabetes as well.

By now, we can rattle off facts and figures about the disease in our sleep. Of course, knowing how insulin shots work doesn't make us wish one bit less for the day a cure is found and the shots are obsolete. Knowing what causes diabetic complications doesn't make them any less frightening. But we have found that learning as much about diabetes as we can helps us feel much less helpless. Diabetes is one of the few serious diseases in which the patient's knowledge and behavior can have a significant impact on the course the disease takes. It's one of the few conditions that puts *you* in the driver's seat. There are a great many things you and your child can do to lessen the impact diabetes has on her health and her life, and understanding the disease is the first step toward controlling it.

Diabetes is a leading cause of death in the United States and a major contributor to heart disease, which is our nation's number-one killer. The disease costs this nation about $20 billion a year in medical costs and lost work time, and the figure's rising fast. So is the number of people who *have* diabetes. Though scientists are unsure why, more children have diabetes today than ever before. If your child is one of them, you'll want to know as much as possible about insulin-dependent diabetes mellitus (IDDM).

Scientists are still looking for a more precise explanation of how and why diabetes develops, but the most widely accepted hypothesis today is that in Type-I diabetics, the body's defense system actually destroys the islet cells that produce insulin. IDDM is an auto-immune disease—a disease in which instead of just protecting the body from foreign "invaders," like viruses, the body's immune system malfunctions and also attacks the body's own cells, giving whole new meaning to the phrase "self-destructive behavior."

Though diabetes is usually acutely set off by a trigger (chicken pox was the suspected culprit for Casey), the trigger doesn't *cause* the disease. To develop diabetes, you must be genetically predisposed to it. The fact that fewer than 8 percent of diabetics' siblings develop diabetes suggests that the hereditary process is far more complicated than the one that governs eye color or other genetic conditions such as hemophilia or color blindness. Today, through research to prevent and cure diabetes, scientists are developing a greater understanding of just *how* diabetes is transmitted.

While scientists are still learning about how diabetes develops and passes from one generation to the next, they're already pretty knowledgeable about how the disease affects the human body. Diabetes is more than simply "high blood sugar." Yes, diabetics do have too much sugar in their blood, but it's not necessarily because they eat too much sugar. Rather, the Type-I diabetic's pancreas fails to produce insulin, the hormone that metabolizes food into usable energy.

If you were to eavesdrop on a bunch of dieters bemoaning their fat thighs, you'd likely hear at least one blame her chubbiness on a "slow metabolism." But metabolism is not a magic process that turns a six-course lunch into a size-six figure. It's the biological mechanism that converts food into energy.

Healthy bodies use insulin to metabolize glucose, which turns it into energy the body can use. Much of the food we eat turns to sugar that then must be converted to energy. When the pancreas fails to produce enough insulin (or any at all), the sugar remains unused and is excreted in the urine. The energy from food goes to waste, and the body becomes deprived of the energy it needs to function.

There are two kinds of diabetes: Type-I, or insulin-dependent diabetes mellitus (IDDM) and Type-II, commonly known as adult-onset diabetes. IDDM affects about 10 to 15 percent of all diabetics, and is more serious and harder to handle than adult-onset diabetes. For while Type-II diabetes can sometimes be treated with diet and oral medication alone, Type-I diabetics must take insulin shots to stay alive.

Injected insulin does not *cure* diabetes. It just helps the body function more normally. Before the discovery of insulin therapy in the 1920s, the life expectancy of a child with diabetes was about two years after the diagnosis. But today, thanks to insulin, many diabetics who were diagnosed as children are now in their seventies.

One common misconception about diabetes is that if

the disease is caused by too much undigested sugar in the blood, it can be cured by eliminating sugary foods like cake and candy. The problem with this assumption is that even foods that don't taste "sugary" break down into sugars. This is especially true of starches, or complex carbohydrates. A perfect example of this process is the ripening of a banana. When a banana is just picked, it may taste mealy and have a starchy or potato-like texture. As it ripens, the starch breaks down into sugar. That's why older bananas taste sweeter. In your body, digestive enzymes do to starches what time does to bananas: breaks them down into sugars. If you were to eliminate from your diet every food that broke down into glucose, you'd have to subsist on celery and water.

When the pancreas doesn't produce insulin (as is the case in Type-I diabetes) or doesn't utilize it properly (in Type-II), the assembly line breaks down midpoint. Starches and complex sugars are broken down into glucose, but the body is unable to convert that glucose into energy. Having nowhere to go, the glucose piles up, unused, in the body.

If left unchecked, hyperglycemia (high blood sugar) can result in a coma. Since the body can't use its sugar for energy, it "borrows" from fat stores, and the body releases ketones, which are poisonous. If ketoacidosis (as this state is called) continues, the patient may ultimately lapse into a coma. The symptoms of impending diabetic coma can include foul, or "sweet," breath (the smell comes from the ketones), excessive thirst, or fatigue.

Those of us who have dieted to lose the five pounds we gained on a vacation may be used to the philosophy that if reducing caloric intake by 100 calories a day is good, reducing it by 200 is better; if a hundred sit-ups are good, two hundred are better. This kind of thinking is not only inaccurate when it comes to diabetes, but potentially dangerous. If your child eats too little or exercises too much relative to the amount of insulin she's injected, she can go into an insulin reaction. Symptoms include profuse sweating, weakness, rapid pulse, pale clammy skin, trembling, or crankiness (the same kind of low-sugar mood that might strike you on a day you were too busy to eat lunch). Over time, this type of blood-sugar swing, or swings to the other extreme of *hyper*-glycemia, can lead to complications. But exercising and maintaining blood-glucose levels at a healthy level can greatly lessen the likelihood of those complications developing as your child gets older. Because these are achievable goals (or goals you can come very close to) you *can* make a difference in the path your child's diabetes takes.

Although diabetes is a disease of one small body organ, its complications can affect the entire body. Diabetics can go blind, lose kidney function, and need to have their limbs amputated due to circulatory problems. They are more susceptible to problems ranging from gum disease to heart disease, develop more bodily infections than the average person, and recover from these infections much more slowly. But these complications *can* be minimized with proper blood-sugar control and with treatment of minor problems before they get out of hand. Therefore, if you understand the complications clearly and know exactly what you're up against, you can take steps to safeguard your child's health.

Thanks to scientific advances, complications are much easier to prevent than ever before. So try to focus on the positives — your ability to control diabetes — rather than the negative of the complications themselves. That way, instead of walking around burdened by anxiety, you can operate from a position of strength, buoyed by the knowledge that with vigilance and care you *can* help your child prevent (or at least significantly lessen) diabetes's complications. It's also important to focus on your child's capabilities rather than on her limitations. Remember that the psychological risks of overprotecting your child often exceed the physical risks you're protecting her from.

Because a known enemy is more easily conquered, following is an outline of some diabetes complications:

Diabetes can cause and aggravate dental problems (and dental problems can, in turn, complicate diabetes). The glucose in diabetic blood lingers in the mouth and leads to plaque and bacteria, just as drinking lots of fruit punch or chewing lots of sugary gum might for non-diabetics. Furthermore, diabetics' arteries are often partially clogged and the reduction in circulation in the gums' little blood vessels makes healing of minor cuts and mouth sores more difficult.

Diabetics are also at a higher risk than most people for the type of serious gum disease that can make teeth fall out. Interestingly, diabetes doesn't initially cause gum disease. It's just that in diabetics, gum disease is much harder to cure. Therefore, it is important to do whatever possible to make sure gum disease doesn't begin in the first place. Periodontal disease can not only be painful and annoying, but actually can make it harder to control diabetes. Why? Just ask the residents of an old-age home. Sore gums and toothlessness can make eating painful. That makes it harder for diabetics to stick to well-planned eating schedules — and thus makes it almost impossible to control diabetes effectively.

To prevent dental problems, make sure your child is brushing her teeth several times a day — and brushing *properly* (none of the old "one stroke down, one stroke up, and we're done!"). Have your dentist teach her how to floss her teeth properly every day, too, and make frequent appointments for professional teeth cleanings.

Diabetes is the leading cause of new adult blindness in America, with about 6,000 cases reported each year. Even in diabetics who retain their eyesight, about 90 percent will have some changes in the eye's structure after about fifteen years, and diabetics can develop a vision-endangering condition called proliferative diabetic retinopathy after about thirty years of living with Type-I diabetes.

Diabetic retinopathy occurs when the retina, which lines the back of the eye and transmits visual images to the brain, is damaged by the deterioration of the small blood vessels that bring the retina the oxygen it needs. As with many diabetic complications, the root of the problem is poor circulation. Doctors are developing exciting new ways to minimize these risks, and thanks to better blood-sugar control, this condition is far less common than it once was. Today, more than ever, vigilance and proper care can significantly reduce the risk of long-term complications.

Take your child to a licensed ophthalmologist (not an optician or optometrist) at least once a year, and call your doctor immediately if your child experiences any blurred or double vision, pain around or behind the eyes, or "spots" floating in front of her eyes.

Diabetes is literally a head-to-toe disease: Along with dental and ophthalmological complications, diabetes can also lead to serious problems in the feet — problems that, in some cases, make amputation necessary. A diabetic's feet are more vulnerable to infection, because diabetes can cause the blood vessel walls to thicken, which reduces circulation to the lower legs and feet. When circulation is impaired, it takes longer for sores to heal, and makes it easier for infections to develop. The risk of infection is increased, too, by the fact that diabetics often have less acute sensations in their limbs. A diabetic with a cut on her foot may not even feel it until it has become infected.

Like dental problems, foot problems can be minimized by good blood-sugar control and attentive care. The vast majority of the 20,000 foot and leg amputations performed in this country each year can be traced to some degree of neglect. Prevention and attention to minor problems before they become major could help the diabetic population avoid as many as 75 percent of all these devastating procedures.

Proper foot care starts with proper shoe selection. Don't wait until your child notices that her shoes are too tight before replacing them with a larger size. Develop a rapport with a shoe-store salesman you like and take your child in for frequent fittings. Make sure shoes have adequate toe room and do not cause rubs or blisters anywhere. Diabetics should wear shoes at all times to avoid tiny cuts and splinters that can become infected. Socks are also important, so shop for ones that *breathe* (no nylon, please!).

Treat your child's feet with tender-loving care, using lots of moisturizer when they're dry and plenty of moisture-absorbing talc when they're sweaty. Use sunblock to avoid burns that can lead to peeling; tops of feet are one of the most frequently forgotten sunburn zones. Cut toenails carefully, straight across, and for goodness' sake, don't treat your child's calluses or corns yourself. Your pediatrician is probably not a pro at diabetic foot care, either. Ask your diabetes specialist to recommend a podiatrist or specially trained nurse.

Inspect your child's feet every night. With little children, this can be done in a non-threatening round of "This little piggy went to market." (Somehow we doubt you'll get your fifteen-year-old to sit through that!) Swelling, change in color, or change in the texture of the foot's skin can signal an infection brewing, as can a bad odor. Encourage your child to start examining her own feet as soon as she's old enough, and it ultimately will become as much a part of her pre-bedtime routine as teeth-brushing and face-washing.

Another major complication of diabetes is kidney disease, or nephropathy. Up to 40 percent of insulin-dependent diabetics develop some sort of kidney problems when they're adults, making kidney disease 500 times more common in adults with insulin-dependent diabetes mellitus than in the general population.

In diabetic nephropathy, the kidneys overwork to filter out the excess sugar in the blood. It is filtered into the urine, which is "manufactured" in the kidneys. This is why, in the old days, diabetics monitored their glucose levels by checking their urine. As the small vessels in the kidneys become damaged from overuse, scar tissue builds up, and makes it impossible for the kidneys to work efficiently. In the worst-case scenario, the kidneys stop functioning altogether and the body is poisoned by its own waste.

New drugs and changes in diet can slow kidney deterioration, and new tests for microalbumen in the urine can help identify kidney disease very early. The risk is much smaller than it once was, but it's still very important to watch for signs of kidney trouble and treat them immediately.

Be sure to alert your doctor if your child suffers from a urinary tract infection (often characterized by painful urination) or receives a blow to the kidneys. That can happen in rough-and-tumble sports or even if your child lands with a bump during a sleigh ride. Don't panic, though; even when it happens, it rarely causes a problem.

Like most other diabetic complications, kidney problems can be minimized by careful control of blood glucose, which lightens the kidneys' filtering load. Controlling blood pressure is also important. High blood pressure can weaken blood vessels even more and can speed damage. Make sure your doctor checks your child's blood pressure at every visit and compares the readings with age-normal values. Regular exercise, which keeps blood moving through the body's veins and arteries, is one of the best and easiest ways to control both blood pressure and blood-glucose levels.

Diabetes can also lead to nerve disease, or neuropathy. In fact, detectable loss of nerve function occurs in approximately 40 percent of all diabetics. But when your child controls her blood glucose and follows her doctor's prescriptions for exercise, diet, and insulin doses, the risks of diabetic neuropathy are greatly minimized.

Again, the key is knowing what symptoms spell trouble. Contact your doctor for help if your child experiences "pins and needles" (like the feeling that your foot's asleep, which most healthy adults experience from time to time), frequent itching, or other abnormal sensations. Often, these symptoms appear as an initial reaction to insulin and disappear once the body gets used to the hormone injections. Keep track of the responses, but don't panic if you notice them soon after your child is diagnosed and starts treatment.

The poor circulation that causes many of the problems listed above can also lead to heart trouble. Diabetes is a major cause of heart disease, which is itself the number-one killer in America. Doctors are currently studying the ways diabetes thickens blood-vessel walls. They already know for sure that the clogging of a diabetic's arteries can decrease circulation and necessitate the heart's having to pump harder.

That's just one reason diet and exercise are so vital to diabetics. Eating well, exercising frequently, and controlling blood-sugar levels over a lifetime minimizes the risk of cardiac complications and other problems associated with diabetes. Remember that a heart-smart diet never hurt anybody. In fact, many parents of diabetics note that they themselves lose weight and get healthier once the family's kitchen is converted from "junk-food central" to a healthy haven.

The person who invented the slogan, "An ounce of prevention is worth a pound of cure (or treatment)" was surely a diabetic. Monitoring blood sugar and responding to the highs and lows you discover *before* they become problematic can make the difference between a life of illness and anxiety and a life that is happy, relatively healthy, and filled with hope for the future.

Remember: Though it's impossible for a diabetic to have perfect blood-sugar levels every day, you and your child *can* control her blood sugar to a great extent, and you can minimize the risk of complications. All you need are the three "Cs": Confidence, Care, and Control.

5

Diabetes Control:
The Juggling Act

Diabetes is a complicated disease that must be treated by a physician. The facts and advice in this chapter are intended for informational purposes only, and should never replace proper medical care. The authors, contributors, and publishers cannot accept any liability for the consequences of use — or misuse — of this information.

When we brought Casey home from the hospital, we felt exactly as we had when we brought her home as a newborn — except without the glee. We were incredibly nervous about doing things right. At the beginning, we were on the phone to Dr. Ginsberg three times a day. Every time we tested Casey's blood, we'd call the doctor, and say, "Her blood was such and such and this is what she's done today," and we'd find out how much insulin to inject.

Even with that constant contact with our doctor, Casey's blood sugar went very low at school a couple of times in the weeks following her hospitalization, and she almost fainted because her doses weren't yet fine-tuned to her school-day activity schedule.

Our experience seems to be the rule rather than the exception. Although most diabetics have good blood-sugar control in the hospital, many face challenges when they go home to their routine — or more accurately, the *lack* of routine that's so much a part of our lives. By the time we got Casey's insulin doses matched to her school schedule, it was summer vacation time, and Casey's schedule changed again, necessitating even more insulin changes.

At first, achieving the balance between your child's calorie intake and expenditures and her insulin needs may seem like a frustrating drill in trying to center a framed photograph on the wall: "Too high," says the observer, so you lower the picture. "Too low," comes the response, so you raise it again, trying to zero in on exactly the right spot. Newly diagnosed diabetics often find that it takes a while to find out *how much* exercise will keep glucose stable. If they run around too much, glucose levels dip. *How many* carbohydrates must they eat to maintain equilibrium? If they eat too much, glucose levels soar. *How often* should insulin be given? What works today may not be right tomorrow. Your doctor will give you guidelines for all of these factors, and you will undoubtedly have to adjust those guidelines a few times. The changes are compounded by what's known as a "honeymoon phase." During this period, which generally lasts a few weeks to several months (depending on how long your child was acutely diabetic before she was diagnosed), the pancreas gives a "last-hurrah" performance, producing its own insulin and decreasing the amount that needs to be injected. After the honeymoon is over and the beta cells stop producing insulin altogether, your child will probably need more insulin.

Ultimately, your child's insulin needs will stabilize somewhat, though they will continue to vary to some degree throughout her life. Don't worry. You'll soon develop pretty sharp instincts about controlling your child's diabetes and knowing what situations require a doctor's intervention and which you can handle on your own.

"Ultimately," says Dr. Ginsberg, "the goal is for the patient to be the doctor. After all, you have to live with diabetes twenty-four hours a day, and nobody has a live-in doctor. Parents have got to learn for themselves how to keep their child's blood-glucose levels in control."

The key to maintaining that close control is keeping careful track of your child's blood-glucose levels, and responding to them with the appropriate changes in diet, insulin doses, and exercise. Until about ten years ago, all diabetics monitored the sugar-level in their urine. Today, though, most doctors recognize that this makes about as much sense as locking the barn door after the horses have all been stolen. By the time glucose is excreted in the urine, it has been lingering in the bloodstream for hours. Monitoring blood-sugar levels directly with *blood* tests is more effective and efficient. The more accurate readings — and the patient's ability to make changes based on these readings — have gone a long way in helping diabetics avoid the glucose fluctuations that can contribute to long-term complications.

Monitoring is important even for diabetics on a closely controlled plan of insulin, diet, and exercise, because blood-sugar balance can respond to outside factors like illnesses as minor as the flu and stress. Test extra-carefully around exam time or at other stressful periods, like the few days before a new school year or a class play. The testing takes all of about forty-five seconds and is simple. Casey has been doing it herself since she was nine.

Your doctor or diabetes educator will teach you how to do

a blood-glucose check, but here's a basic rundown:

First, wash your hands in warm water, if possible. The warm water helps bring blood to the surface, and makes it easier to do the test.

Second, prick the index, middle, or ring finger. (The thumb is too flat and therefore its blood tends to form a smear instead of a droplet.) Be sure to push the lancet hard enough to draw blood the first time. The tendency is to push gently, but the soft stabs hurt just as much — and you might end up poking ten times without drawing blood if you don't use enough pressure.

Then, squeeze the finger gently from the base up to the tip, "milking" a drop of blood to the pinprick site. Touch the droplet of blood to a test strip, and insert the strip into the meter. Do not touch the finger, as this tends to smear the blood, which confuses the test meter.

Some test kits will give you a digital reading, and others have color-coded charts like those at-home pregnancy tests that advertise "pink means yes, blue means no," and the test strips turn colors depending on the glucose levels.

Make sure to test your glucose monitor periodically against either a back-up monitor in your home or a monitor in your doctor's office. Like all machines, glucose monitors sometimes malfunction. Checking them periodically reduces the chances that your child is walking around with high or low blood sugar while you are getting "normal" readings.

Your doctor will tell you what readings she finds acceptable. In general, 80 to 120 mg is considered normal in non-diabetic children, but trying to keep a young child's sugar levels within these limits often leads to readings of 40 or 400, says Dr. Ginsberg. It is usually better to aim for 100 to 150 or even as high as 180.

"I wish I had realized sooner that swings in blood sugar are normal," says Ellen Smith, a mother who says managing diabetes has gotten easier for her and her family over time. "You can be doing everything perfectly and the readings may still be erratic. Rather than letting these minor fluctuations upset me, I've started concentrating more on the hemoglobin A1C test than on the day-to-day values."

The A1C test lets your doctor see not only what your child's blood-sugar level is on the day the test is administered, but what it has been overall for the past several months. If your child's glucose readings are frequently high and/or the A1C test indicates a problem, the doctor will talk to you about adjusting your child's diet, insulin, exercise — or all three. But if you suspect a problem, don't wait for a quarterly checkup to discuss it. Call your doctor and ask whether she wants you to change something in your child's insulin dose or schedule. That's what she's there for!

Before we discuss *injecting* insulin, let's clarify a few things about what it is and how it works. Insulin is not a drug or a medicine. It is a hormone produced by healthy bodies that diabetics need to supply artificially. In healthy bodies, insulin is produced in beta cells in the pancreas, which is a gland located behind the stomach. The body produces a low level of insulin all the time and a burst of the hormone after meals (just as you do a routine housecleaning every week and a blitz after your teenager is home alone all week).

Without insulin, the diabetic's body can't metabolize glucose and bring it to the cells. Unlike other compounds that can be ingested orally (like lactase for those who have trouble digesting milk products) the diabetic's body is its own worst enemy when it comes to digesting glucose. Insulin can't be ingested like food. The body's digestive system will destroy it.

Injectable insulin, once derived solely from cows and pigs, is now more frequently made in a laboratory by genetic engineers and is virtually identical to normal human insulin. Because animal-derived insulins (which are used less and less, these days) are not exactly the same as that produced in humans, some people are actually allergic to those insulins, and develop a rash or irritation at the injection site. These reactions, though usually harmless and short-lived, should be reported to your physician nonetheless. If the allergy persists, your child may need to be desensitized to the insulin by starting with a very low dose and building up to the amount her body actually requires. The body gets used to the insulin slowly, just as you get used to cold swimming-pool water as you inch your way into the deeper end.

As scientists develop a better understanding of how insulin works, they have developed types of insulin that work *better,* with different types of insulin being used for different periods of time.

• Rapid, or regular activity insulin starts working within half an hour of injection, and works most efficiently in the period within one to four hours after administration. Rapid insulin remains in the bloodstream for eight to sixteen hours, depending on the injection sites used, the individual child, and the type of physical activity being done. Because of the rapidity with which these kinds of insulin work, they're ideal for times when blood sugar is excessively high. Increasingly, rapid-acting insulins are used in combination with longer-lasting formulas to give the body both the "immediate action" it needs and the longer-term stability of slower-acting insulin.

• Intermediate action insulin (also called NPH or lente) reaches the bloodstream an hour and a half to two hours after injection, peaks six to ten hours later, and lasts about a day.

• Long-acting or ultralente insulins take four to six hours to start working; as such, they are inappropriate for use when the body needs insulin quickly. Long-acting insulin lasts about a day and a half (though its effectiveness lessens considerably over time), and is generally reserved for older patients with erratic schedules. Ultralente insulin must be supplemented with regular insulin before meals, as must intermediate action insulin.

No one type of insulin is right for every person, or every situation. Your doctor will prescribe an insulin regime based on a number of factors including your child's physiology, her schedule and yours, and the balance of eating and exercising.

Insulin dosages are measured in units. The more units of insulin your child injects, the greater its effect on lowering blood-glucose levels. "U-100," the standard syringe capacity, means there are 100 units of insulin in each cubic centimeter (cc or ml) of the liquid. A child who requires more insulin does not necessarily have "worse" diabetes than one who needs less. Insulin doses have more to do with body size, exercise level, and diet than with the "severity" of diabetes.

Though refrigerating insulin isn't strictly necessary (except in tropical climates), keeping extra insulin bottles in the refrigerator not only keeps them at a constant temperature as the weather changes but, on a more practical level, assures they're always in exactly the same place when the old bottle is finished and it's time to start a new one. (Imagine how much easier life would be if we all kept our car keys in the fridge. We figure it would save about thirty-five minutes a week in turning-over-the-house time!) The bottle you're currently using should be kept in a cool — but not cold — place.

Like milk, insulin comes with an "expiration date." Do *not* use expired insulin (except in dire emergencies), because as it starts to lose its effectiveness, it can throw off your careful calculations of how much is needed.

Because measuring insulin sometimes requires a knowledge of fractions — and because she's a little squeamish — Casey didn't initially like to do her own shots. While it's important to encourage your child to become independent, you've also got to take into account that young children may not really be able to measure and inject their own insulin. For a while, then, the shots will be up to you.

"Before we send patients home," explains Paula Liguori, our nurse-educator, "we make sure the parents have practiced giving shots to themselves and each other, so that they know that the shot isn't all that painful. We never use oranges or grapefruits, because while that may teach you the technique, we think it's critical for parents to understand what it feels like to get an insulin shot, and to develop some empathy for what their child is going through."

Your doctor or diabetes educator will teach *you* how to give an injection, and will review the procedures with you until you're comfortable with them. But here, for handy reference, are a few things you need to know about injecting insulin, along with some advice about making shot time easier.

• Anyone giving an injection for the first time (or the hundredth, for that matter) is worried about air bubbles. We've all heard horror stories about what happens if a tiny bubble gets into the vein. Luckily, insulin is injected *not* into veins or muscles, but into subcutaneous tissue—the layer right beneath the fat. While it's best that there be no air bubbles in the syringe because they take up space that should be filled with insulin for precise dosage, you needn't panic about injecting a bubble or two. It's harmless.

• If some insulin drips out of the syringe, don't try to make it up in approximate measure; you're likely to over-inject. If you've lost just a drop, don't worry. If you've lost more than that, call your doctor.

• Rotate the site of injections. Otherwise, skin may thicken and make it harder to give injections. Plus, the thickening can be unsightly, and the last thing a diabetic child needs is another reason to feel different. Some doctors suggest a rigid site-rotation program: Monday: right arm; Tuesday: left arm. Our doctor suggests that her patients rotate their injection sites based on how rapidly the insulin absorbs from different places in the body. "Shots given into the abdomen are absorbed most quickly," explains Dr. Ginsberg. "So that's where we recommend shots if a child's blood glucose level is high. The arm is the next fastest absorbing site, followed by the leg and the buttocks. Rotating sites based on blood-sugar levels may be a bit more complicated than following a strict rotation, but it also allows for better blood-glucose control."

Of course, you can only rotate the shots to those body sites with enough tissue to absorb the insulin. For a long time Casey was so thin that we could only give her shots in her backside. We couldn't inject her arm, because no matter where we stuck the needle, she'd bleed. We couldn't give her her shots in her thigh, for the same reason. Once she put on some weight we started rotating her sites, but since she started giving herself shots, we're facing another challenge: When Casey gives herself her shot, she can only maneuver well enough to do it on one hip, so she doesn't really rotate her sites. Dr. Ginsberg says this is very common, but that diabetics need to be encouraged to find other spots they can inject. "We try to discourage favoring one spot because it can lead to hypertrophy (thickening) of the tissue," says Dr. Ginsberg, "and can also reduce the insulin's effective absorption over time."

• If you are rotating sites but still find you're getting a small lump under the skin after a shot, you're giving the injection too shallowly. If you're having trouble with the technique, review it with your doctor or diabetes educator.

• Make sure you're aiming the needle perpendicularly to the skin (in other words, the skin and the needle should form a plus-sign shape).

• One mother we spoke to recommended putting ice on the injection site to numb the skin a bit before giving the injection. Dr. Ginsberg says this isn't a great long-term idea because it can damage the tissue, but it is a good way to get a newly diagnosed child used to the shots more gradually.

• Don't squeeze the injection site too tightly; this causes pressure in the area, and forces some of the insulin back out.

• The more quickly you give the shot, the less painful it is, the same way that pulling off a Band-Aid quickly stings less than peeling it off s-l-o-w-l-y. The nerve endings where the shot is felt are in the skin. So the sooner you get the needle through that skin to the underlying tissue, the faster the unpleasant part of the shot is over. Think about the last time your own doctor took your blood. You only felt the needle as it was going in and coming out. For the minute or two it was *through* the skin, you probably didn't feel a thing.

Remember that while children with diabetes are no more susceptible than their peers to the usual childhood diseases, in diabetic children minor infections and viruses can affect glucose levels, often elevating them and forming ketones. Do not skip insulin injections when your child is sick with a cold or flu, and — no matter how convincingly she begs you through a haze of germs — don't skip regular glucose testing. It's more important on "sick days" than ever. Many liquid medicines (antibiotics, cough syrups, stomachache remedies) have lots of sugar in them. Be aware of this when testing your child's blood on a "sick day" and don't be too alarmed if her sugar is high. If it's over 240 mg/dl, test the urine for ketones.

Make sure your child is drinking plenty of fluids. If she's eating her usual diet, the extra fluids should be sugar-free. But if her flu or virus has left her with no appetite, make sure the fluids replace the calories she needs. Apple juice, Gatorade, and grape juice are all high in calories, and are good choices when your child isn't eating anything else. We gave Casey popsicles when she had a stomach virus and was too sick to eat. They supplied enough calories and she loved it.

Call your specialist if your child is on any medication or if you have any questions about sick-day procedures, and make sure that you follow her instructions about insulin doses and injections.

To make the injection-giving easier (when your child is

otherwise healthy, as well as when she's sick) you may want to take advantage of some of the new technology to make shot times easier, too. Several companies manufacture injection aids, which help you get the needle in at the correct angle. The aid cloaks the needle, and holds the skin taut for injection, shooting the needle in quickly. While it is completely possible to give a perfect shot without one of these devices, you might want to try one if the needle-hiding aspect will make shot-time easier on you and your child. Sale never used one when injecting Casey's insulin, but Casey herself liked to use them when she started doing her own shots.

Standard syringes are no longer the only way to inject insulin. Today, diabetes equipment companies offer pens that are pre-loaded and inject the insulin with one click of a button. There are also long-acting pumps that introduce insulin into the body in a slow trickle all day long. An insulin pen, which looks like a fountain pen and is filled with regular insulin cartridges, can make pre-meal shots less complicated. The pens are adjustable, to vary the amount of insulin injected. The pens' needles are so fine, many patients find that shots given with insulin pens are less painful than those given by traditional syringe.

Infusers, which keep a line open in the skin for injections, may make the process easier, too—think of it as an "open phone line" to your child's blood stream.

Jet injectors, which are needle free, deliver insulin by spraying insulin through the skin at high pressure. These are not entirely pain-free, and because they are rather cumbersome, jet infusers are not often recommended for children.

Researchers are currently trying to figure out ways to make insulin "nasal sprays." Because the inside of the nose is lined with mucous membrane, it's good at conducting things into the blood stream. The technology is not yet available, but it's yet another example of the ways doctors are working to make life easier for diabetic children. Ask your doctor which method will work best for you.

There's no question that diabetes science is advancing, and both the insulins and the "tools of the trade" are getting better all the time. But until a cure is found, diabetics will always have to do a bit of juggling. Your doctor will give you specific prescriptions for your child's diet as she has for the insulin dosages. What follows is just a basic review of how the exchange system works and how exercise can help control blood-sugar levels.

If you've ever been on a Weight Watchers–type diet, the diabetic diet's exchange lists that your doctor gives you will seem familiar. Your child's doctor or dietitian will prescribe a daily allotment of "bread exchanges," "meat exchanges," "dairy exchanges," and so on. You and your child will plan menus based on the number of servings specified for each meal and each snack. Now that the FDA is becoming stricter about food labeling, you can find out how many grams of fat, protein, and carbohydrates are in most of the foods you see on the supermarket shelves. This will help you determine what store-bought foods give you the number of carbohydrates, protein, fat, and calories recommended by your doctor or dietitian.

As Lynne W. Scott, M.A., R.D./L.D., explains, "Exchange lists are averages used for groups of food. They are an easy way of classifying food so that the diabetic can have a well-balanced diet." Scott, who is co-author of *The Living Heart Diet* and *The Living Heart Brand-Name Shopper's Guide,* stresses that it's important to monitor not only the number of servings your child eats, but the type of fat in each food. The amount of saturated fat (primarily animal fat) should be low because diabetics are at increased risk of heart disease.

But don't worry too much about feeding your child "perfect" meals. "Don't force your child to eat anything she hates," says Dr. Ginsberg, "because this just turns food into a battle ground, and it really isn't necessary for diabetes control."

"It's important to stick to the diet your physician and dietitian have developed for your child," Scott says, "but it's also important to be realistic. The goal is for your child to get enough calories for growth and development."

Part of this "realism" is accepting the fact that kids are faced with dozens of temptations every day—at school, at birthday parties, and at friends' houses. "The hardest part for kids," Scott says, "is to see what other kids are eating." To make that easier, all of the parents we interviewed agreed: Talk to your dietitian about handling special events like birthday parties and holidays, and never say "never"; rather, show your child how to accommodate her exercise and insulin to what she's eating. "I tell my son to bring his treats from parties or Halloween home," says Susan Briston. "We save them and fit them in as his snacks or the extra food he needs during sports. By not saying he can never eat these foods, I make sure he isn't constantly craving them, which could set him up for a binge."

Of course, learning how to balance food and exercise may take your child some time. After all, how many six-year-olds understand what a calorie is, or have the mathematical ability to multiply grams times calories. But there are things you can do to teach your child responsibility for her diet, starting at an early age.

With children ages six and seven, explains Lynne Scott, the mother usually is still responsible for what the child eats. At this stage, you can teach a child which foods are part of each exchange group. As they get older, they can learn to measure how much mashed potatoes is a half a cup, which equals a serving of bread. A little further on, they can learn how to prepare some of their own snacks. Kitchen activity helps your child learn how to "eyeball" food and figure out the exchanges.

In our house, we experiment with snacks and recipes all the time. For example, we'll make banana bread without the sugar. Because bananas are sweet we find that we don't even *miss* the sugar. We've learned to "doctor" recipes so that they're safe for Casey to eat but still taste good, paying careful attention to the guidelines our doctor has set forth. We buy many diabetic cookbooks, and lots of them are inaccurate. They say, "You can eat this and you can eat that . . . " when Casey isn't supposed to eat those things more than once in a very rare while. Every doctor and every dietitian has her own idea about what diets work—and every diabetic's body reacts differently to food. For example, some of the diets you read about for diabetics include lots of fruit, but our doctor said Casey needs to avoid sugar-intense fruits like grapes, peaches, and plums except right before exercise.

We try to find other things she likes to compensate, so she doesn't feel deprived. For example, Casey's snack at school is usually ten potato chips and a glass of milk—food most kids crave. Before she was diagnosed, Casey was never allowed to have soda. Now we let her have diet soda as a treat. As you start adapting to your child's new diet, you'll probably find that you give your child special treats, too, because there are so many things your child *can't* eat. Overall, the diabetic diet is a very healthful one, and it's a diet you can *live* with (both literally and figuratively). We try to have our whole family follow it.

Besides following your doctor's prescriptions for *what* your child can eat, it's important to attend to the "when." Doctors generally recommend that meals are eaten when insulin is at its peak (about half an hour after injection). So when we're eating out in a restaurant, we make sure not to give Casey her shot until after we are seated. That way, if our 8 o'clock reservation isn't honored till 8:30 because someone else's dinner is going on forever, we don't have to worry about mistiming the shot.

When you *are* eating in a restaurant, be sure to ask a lot of questions: What's in that sauce? Is the chicken fried or baked? If the waiter is being difficult, just explain that your child is diabetic. When the restaurant staff knows you're not just being a "picky eater," they're usually very accommodating.

But what happens when you're not around to ask the questions or to make sure that your child is using the answers to make responsible decisions?

Accept the fact that you may not be able to control every morsel your child ingests. After all, she's not a machine but a person with likes, dislikes, and moods, just like the rest of us. Young children, for instance, tend to go through food phases: only peanut butter, nothing green. Teenagers often rebel by eating the foods they know they shouldn't. Even when they are not being rebellious, most kids who have had diabetes for a few years pick up on the fact that eating a forbidden food isn't going to make them sick—at least, it's not going to give them symptoms they can see or feel—so they tend to put the dangers out of their minds and give into the cravings and peer pressure.

When Casey eats sugary foods that aren't good for her she doesn't feel sick. Unless her blood sugar were to go *really* high, she might not feel anything at all, though the hyperglycemia can do damage to cell tissue over time. But if she takes too much insulin and doesn't eat enough, her blood sugar drops and she feels sick. The difference between how immediately noticeable low blood sugar is and how long it takes to actually feel the problem when blood sugar is high, all but psyches many kids to eat more so that they don't go low. It doesn't scare Casey to *overeat* like it scares her to *undereat,* even though it's better for her body if she eats a little less.

If your child is overeating behind your back, she may even cover up her "sneak attacks" by altering her test-result journals. It's important to stress to your child that falling "off the wagon" and admitting it is better than covering it up. In fact, if you can get your child to talk to you about which temptations are hardest for her to pass up, you, the doctor, or the dietitian may be able to help her come up with ways either to resist the temptation by substituting a less sugary food, or by adjusting her exercise schedule to accommodate occasional dietary lapses.

That's one way exercise comes into play, but maintaining a high level of activity is not just a "fixit." It is — or should be — an integral part of every diabetic's life.

Like the rest of our family, Casey was always very active, so getting her on a regular exercise schedule was "no sweat." If your child's favorite sport is changing channels, though, you'll have to be a bit more imaginative. We bought a trampoline for Casey to jump on, and the other kids love it, too. It's great aerobic exercise, and a lot more fun than jumping jacks.

If you and your spouse are couch potatoes, too, why not embark on a family program? Jogging or swimming together is a great way to build not only muscles and endurance, but family closeness, as well.

You might want to keep a few exercise videos on hand for those weeks of endless rain that plague almost every region of this continent. Recreational athletes can afford to "call" a few games on account of rain, but diabetics must try to keep to a pretty regular and active schedule of activity.

Can too much of a good thing be too much? Only if you don't balance your child's exercise, insulin, and diet. Remember that when your child is exercising heavily (on a skiing vacation, or in day camp) you have to beware of the "day-after syndrome." The blood-sugar-lowering effect may occur as late as the next day, and may last up to a full day after the strenuous exercise. During periods of strenuous exercise be sure your child is testing her blood frequently.

"You can be a marathon runner," says Dr. Ginsberg, "but you have to explain to your doctor not only *that* you exercise, but *when, how,* and *at what intensity level.* Last year," she relates, "we had our first experience with a diabetic ballerina. It took us a while to figure out how to control her diabetes, because a dancer's schedule is so unusual. They wake up and exercise all day, and then eat a big meal at midnight, after their performance. We figured out that the best way to keep her glucose levels controlled was usually with just one shot a day, at midnight—a regime very unlike those of our other patients." To illustrate how exercise affects insulin levels, Dr. Ginsberg told us that when the dancer had a one-month vacation and stopped her rehearsal and performance schedule, she needed six times as much insulin as she had before.

So if your child *does* exercise, make sure your doctor knows the nitty-gritty details of her workout — not only how many days a week your daughter goes to a dance class, but whether she actually dances for the full hour or does three pliés at the barre and goes home. Does your soccer player run around the field — or play goalie? Does you teenager follow along with that Jane Fonda videotape, or just sort of watch it? There are no right or wrong answers to these questions — just accurate ones. Giving your doctor the most thorough profile of what your child's life is like will make it much easier for her to prescribe the most effective insulin schedule and diet. Because the amount of exercise your child does — like her diet and adherence to insulin schedules — will affect her health, it is important to be as frank and realistic with your doctor as possible.

We'd all love to claim that our families eat and exercise with clockwork regularity, but in these days of two-career families and increasingly hectic schedules, how many of us can? Save the perfect-family show for your mother-in-law and level with your doctor.

Working closely and honestly with your doctor will help control your child's diabetes, but, unfortunately, even if your child is exercising regularly, eating the right things, and following your doctor's prescriptions for insulin dosages and timing — she will eventually have an insulin reaction. They're almost unavoidable. No matter how well-prepared you are — both practically and emotionally — for an insulin reaction, it's hard not to let the first one (and even the tenth!) throw you.

It's especially common for parents of newly diagnosed diabetics to feel guilty when their child has high or low sugar reactions, but you might as well learn up front: You can't watch your child twenty-four hours a day.

Unless you have arranged a familial dispensation from Murphy's law, the first of these reactions will undoubtedly come at the least convenient time, in the least comfortable surroundings. The August after Casey was diagnosed, we went on a family vacation to Africa. Imagining that the medical care there wouldn't be quite up to the standards we're used to in New York City, we packed valises full of equipment: syringes, insulin, glucose monitors—we felt just like a traveling drugstore. We watched every morsel of the unfamiliar foods Casey put in her mouth, trying to figure out how many "starches" or "proteins" were in the foods we couldn't pronounce, let alone identify.

One afternoon we went with our adult friends to view the leopard cubs and their parents. We left the kids with the nanny and grandparents and their friends. Casey decided to go for a spin on a motorbike and check out the local animals. After all, who travels all the way to Africa to sit around reading comic books? But because the bike was vibrating, Casey couldn't tell that her sugar levels were dipping. She thought her dizziness was just from the ride. When she got off the bike and started to walk back to the house where we were staying, the others noticed how pale she looked, and then she went limp. Marita, the nanny, called us on the walkie-talkie, and we told her to just give Casey some honey and then wait ten minutes and give her some peanut butter and crackers, and we headed back to the house we were staying in immediately. When we got back, Casey was still in bed, weak, but no longer pale and sweaty—and *almost* as frightened as we were!

The paleness and sweatiness that Casey experienced are among the most common signs of a reaction. Other things to watch out for are:

Weakness
Trembling
Nausea
Irritability
Crying jags
Acting confused or appearing drunk

If you or your child notice any of these symptoms you need to raise the blood-glucose level as fast as possible. A drink of fruit juice usually does the trick, and candy or cake icing (you can buy tubes of icing in the supermarket) work, too. Your child ought to carry some "quick sugar" with her at all times, in case she feels herself going low when she's not around you or your refrigerator full of orange juice. Hard candies are portable, as are the little packets of honey that Casey carries with her.

Remember to give your child regular soda with sugar, *not diet soda,* during an insulin reaction. Because it has no sugar, diet soda is absolutely useless in raising glucose levels back to normal.

If the insulin reaction is severe, or if your child is too small to understand what's happening, you may need to force the food. If you can't get her to eat at all, try rubbing some honey on her gums. It will be converted to glucose in the bloodstream almost immediately. Coping with diabetes in infants and toddlers can be especially tough during an insulin reaction. A two-year-old can't tell you when he feels dizzy and a one-year-old can't understand why it's important to eat *now.*

If you're not sure whether your child is having an insulin reaction, it's better to overreact a bit than to underreact. Even if it turns out your child *isn't* having an emergency, the bit of quick sugar you administer can't hurt. Ignoring a reaction can. We try to keep Casey's glucose monitor with us at all times so that we can tell whether her blood sugar is low when we suspect a problem.

About ten minutes after your child eats the sugar, follow it up with a carbohydrate/protein snack, like a turkey sandwich or peanut-butter-on-cracker. (We use natural peanut butter, because it has less sugar, and no insecticide is sprayed on the peanuts when they're growing.)

In more severe cases of insulin shock, injections of glucagon may be necessary. Glucagon gets glucose into the bloodstream *pronto* and is injected into the backside when a child is not alert enough to eat or drink. If your doctor wants you to have glucagon in your arsenal of diabetes-treating equipment, be sure to get *and fill* a prescription as soon after your child's diagnosis as possible. Keep a bottle at home and have one stored at your child's school for emergencies. Make sure the school nurse and your child's teacher know in what circumstances they should administer glucagon, and how to do so.

Unfortunately, occasional insulin reactions are part of the diabetic's life. But if your child seems to be having a *lot* of hypoglycemic episodes, you need to work more carefully, together, on prevention. Here are some steps your doctor might recommend.

1. Increase the frequency with which your child monitors her blood. Perhaps the frequent episodes follow a pattern of glucose dips. The better you and your child understand her body's glucose flow, the better you can manage it.

2. Have your child eat between-meal snacks. Many small meals over the day go a lot further to maintaining steady glucose levels than the traditional "three square meals," which dump large amounts of glucose into the blood

stream rapidly and then offer no more blood sugar for several hours.

3. Offer a before-bedtime snack if pre-bedtime blood sugar isn't too high. This will keep your child's blood-glucose level at healthy minimums while she sleeps. Nighttime lows can be dangerous. That's why our doctor recommends testing midnight blood-sugar levels at least once a week. Talk to your doctor about which of these solutions she prefers.

If your child does have an insulin reaction while she's sleeping, she probably won't remember anything about it when she awakens. The body tends to compensate for the sleep-time hypoglycemia with a rise in sugar, leaving your child with a headache or stomachache in the morning and a high blood-glucose level. If your child reports frequent morning aches, or seems to remember a lot of bad dreams, its probably a sign that you need to talk to your doctor about pre-bedtime measures you can take to avoid this phenomenon (known as the somyogi effect) and maintain control through the night.

Sale used to check Casey's blood sugar every night between midnight and two while Casey slept, because for a while, she was waking up with blood-sugar readings in the 200s every morning. After checking her night-time glucose every hour, we discovered that Casey was going low during sleep and then rebounding, which is what led to the high blood-sugar readings in the morning.

If you visit your doctor after your child has a hypoglycemic episode, be sure to tell her about it. Insulin reactions can lead to high blood-sugar levels, because the reaction releases stored glucose in the body, which combines with the sugar ingested to counteract the hypoglycemia — it's a sort of rebound effect. Be sure to let your doctor know if an insulin reaction has preceded an office visit. Otherwise, she might think the high blood sugar is caused by too little insulin, when the problem is just the opposite.

If your child *is* having extremely high blood-sugar levels, contact your doctor right away. If you're monitoring frequently and properly, you'll probably be able to spot a problem before it gets out of hand. But if you see any of the signs that preceded your child's diagnosis (excessive drinking and urinating, or cold and dry skin, deep breathing, vomiting, or unconsciousness) call your doctor *immediately*. If left untested, ketoacidosis (the condition in which blood sugar is so high that ketones are excreted) can be very dangerous.

Luckily, children with well-controlled diabetes can usually avoid these distressing extremes of the blood-sugar spectrum. But good control doesn't happen by itself. You've got to put in some time and concentration. Working closely with your diabetes specialist and with your own instincts about your child and her health, you will soon be able to work out a program that helps you and your child keep as healthy and in control as possible. If you're having a hard time getting your child to think past next Monday and motivating her with the abstract pay-off of long-term health, try rewarding her control with some shorter-term rewards. Special treats need not be expensive to reinforce your child's diabetes-smart behavior, and meeting short-term goals will spur your child on to keep up the good work and follow her doctor's recommendations week after week, and month after month. More than ever before, close blood-sugar control isn't just a diabetic's dream, but a realistic, attainable goal.

6

Raising the Diabetic Child

Day to day, the hardest part about coping with a child's diabetes is not the shots or the tests; those things really only affect the child and whoever is helping her with the procedures. Often for the family, the hardest thing is coping with the child's mood swings.

Although not every diabetic experiences mood swings, they are very common and may have a medical origin. When a diabetic's insulin shot is close to peaking, her blood sugar goes down—along with her mood. The problem, actually, isn't so much that the blood sugar is *low,* but that it drops so *fast*—usually because it didn't have enough food to stabilize it.

These mood swings can be particularly difficult to handle because when in the midst of what is sometimes called "a hormonal," most diabetics don't accept the fact that they're behaving irrationally. Like sufferers of other hormonally induced mood swings (like PMS), the diabetic in the midst of a mood swing often doesn't realize what's happening. Have you ever seen the PMS-medicine commercial on TV where the woman screams into the phone "I am *not* cranky!" Well, that's pretty much what it's like—but with a diabetic, the mood swings aren't a once-a-month affair, but a frequent problem.

According to our doctor, mood swings can have several causes: "Part of any diabetic child's mood swing problem is sugar-related," explains Dr. Ginsberg, "but there are other factors that may be involved, and you can't describe every bad mood as a 'sugar.' "

"You have to have a consistent way of dealing with the mood swings," says Dr. Ginsberg, noting that the problem can be even harder to deal with in younger children, because they can't verbalize their feelings or their need for some quick carbohydrates. "If you think the mood is diabetes-related," she says, "check your child's blood sugar. Half the time, with the little ones, you'll find out that they're just cranky. If there is a sugar problem," says the doctor, "take care of it. Otherwise, accept the problem for what it is: a bad mood. Two-year-olds with diabetes have temper tantrums, but so do two-year-olds without the disease."

A California mother we interviewed crystallized this approach very succinctly: "Treat your child as a child first," advises Mrs. Singer. "A mood swing doesn't have to be a blood-sugar problem."

Sometimes it's easier than others for us to take a firm stand on diabetic childrens' moods. After all, they have so many burdens because of their diabetes, it seems harsh to hold them accountable for their hormonal mood swings. Ultimately, we feel it's imperative that we hold Casey up to the same standards of behavior as we do our two other girls. All the parents we spoke to agreed:

"It's hard not to coddle my daughter," explains Nancy S., a mother who has coped with her child's illness for the past ten years, "because my guilt bank is always overdrawn. I know there's no way I could make it up to her for all the pain she's endured. But I think there is something I could do to make it all worse, and that's *not* making her aware that there are consequences to her actions. When she was growing up, our daughter saw her older brothers get punished when they misbehaved, and she knows that's what happens when you do something wrong, so we punish her, too."

"I feel so guilty about my daughter's diabetes that I sometimes let her get away with too much," said another mother who's struggling with the peculiar balancing act of raising a diabetic teenager. Let's face it. Any child will manipulate his parents if he knows he can get away with it. Moreover, when you're sticking needles into your child every day, it's especially easy for your child to use your guilt over this to manipulate you. That's one of the reasons our medical team makes parents take a practice injection. "If the parents know what the shot really feels like," explains Paula Liguori, "they won't feel as guilty about giving it."

Diabetic kids learn quickly that dinner time can be a great time to manipulate parents, too, says psychotherapist Maryann Feldstein, who does a lot of work with families of chronically ill children. " 'If you don't buy me that toy,' they threaten, 'I won't eat my dinner.' " Don't fall into the trap, though. A little firmness will benefit your child in the long run.

"By showing our child that she *can't* twist us around her finger in that way," says Nancy S., "by showing her that there are consequences for her actions, we made our daughter realize that we, her parents, are going to be consistent with her and our other kids. If we didn't, we'd have a maniac on our hands. Not only that, we'd have a child who is truly handicapped, because she would lack the skills to get along in the world."

Many of the parents we interviewed told us that not overprotecting their children is one of the hardest parts of raising a diabetic youngster. Like Nancy S. and the other parents we spoke to, experts agree that giving your child room to be a kid is critical to his or her well-being. "Children over-protected in elementary school may have difficulty with social skills, like building friendships," warned Lawrence Kutner, in one of his weekly "Parent & Child" columns in the *New York Times* in the spring of 1991. "They may not know how to handle teasing or other verbal banter and rough play by their classmates. Unless these children develop these skills, they could have difficulty with social relationships."

If this last paragraph alarmed you, please read it again, more carefully. The danger isn't inherent in the diabetes, but in the overprotection that often accompanies the disease. Rearing a diabetic child is fraught with challenges, but so is raising *any* child. The challenges we all face as parents of diabetics are easier to meet when we remember to maintain our perspective and treat our children as normally as possible.

Remember that children — even chronically ill children — are generally pretty flexible, and can adapt to tough life situations like diabetes. We were amazed at first how quickly Casey got into her routine. Even as her parents, we were impressed with how she dealt with all the shots and needles and the blood testing and the routine and the food.

But it became clearer and clearer to us as we were writing this book how very different some of our own perceptions are from Casey's. Sometimes it's tough to remember that children see things in their own way, and that the view is often different — and clearer — on the other side of the syringe.

So talk openly with your child about her feelings, and then use those feelings as your guidelines in developing a coping strategy that's appropriate to your child's age and personality. Of course, your child's perceptions and level of understanding are as individual as her fingerprints, but following are some developmental guidelines that psychologists generally agree might affect your child's reaction to her diabetes.

In an odd way, children who have diabetes from infancy cope with the illness better than children diagnosed later in life, because diabetes is the only life they've ever known. By the time they're old enough to start questioning "Why me?" they are, at least, used to the needles, the diet, the blood tests. But rearing a diabetic infant can be terribly stressful on parents. "The hardest part," says one mother we interviewed, "is not knowing how he's feeling. We have to test his blood sugar constantly, so that we can avoid a low-sugar problem."

If you have a diabetic infant, you can expect her to develop at a normal rate. Diabetes is not a developmental disorder, and your child should start eating, sitting, and walking at the same age she would if healthy. But don't be surprised if your baby takes a few steps back developmentally right after she's diagnosed and hospitalized. Psychological data show that hospitalization in young children can cause regression. A child who drank from a cup may go back to a bottle and one who has just begun to walk may temporarily "forget" how to. Once your baby is back home, she'll regain her ground, but because it's so difficult to communicate with infants and toddlers about their physical and emotional feelings, your diabetic baby will need a lot of attention, explanation, and reassurance.

It's difficult for a preschooler to understand why she needs "medicine" when she feels fine. Emphasize that the insulin is what *keeps* her feeling fine. Don't say, "It will make you better." (Not only because this isn't true, since insulin isn't a cure, but also because it's at odds with a small child's understanding.)

During the preschool years children know that a doctor or parent coming at them with a needle usually means impending pain. It is difficult for them to understand that this "pain" is actually part of something helpful. The same self-centered view of the world that makes preschoolers believe that the moon is shining outside *their* window and that the sun rises because *they* need light makes them believe that their illness is a punishment for some imagined wrongdoing. So try not to reinforce this by scolding your child for moving while getting her fingers stuck, or for trying to avoid an injection. Instead, lavish praise when she holds still or cooperates.

Make sure your child doesn't equate having "good" blood-sugar levels with *being* good. Be careful to describe sugar levels as "high" and "low," not "good" and "bad," says Paula Liguori, otherwise your child will internalize a message that she's bad even when she's stuck to her regime perfectly and blood-sugar levels are high or low for an extraneous reason like stress or an unexpected change in her activity level.

To make shot time easier, reinforce positive behavior rather than dwelling on the negative. "If you place a value on your child's blood-sugar level, you can really damage her self-esteem," says Paula Liguori. "And the damage from that can be worse than a little fluctuation in the sugar." One mother of a nine-year-old, who has been diabetic since in-

fancy, told us that "The biggest challenge in raising a diabetic child is the same as with any child: making sure they
grow up with a positive self-image."

Focusing too closely on your child's blood-sugar levels, or
relating to him as a number can make this a whole lot
tougher, says Paula Liguori. "Many parents use the word
'score' when describing their child's levels, and we always
discourage that approach. This isn't an I.Q. test or S.A.T. It's
not a value measure."

As concerned as you are about your child's health, don't
make her — or yourself — nuts in your quest for "perfect"
blood sugars, or by focusing too intently on the complications that may arise down the line. This can only backfire.
As author Sula Wolf explains in *Children Under Stress:*
"The more anxious the child is about his illness and his
future and the more guilty he feels, the more likely he is to
throw caution to the winds, to flaunt all dietary restrictions
and to be aggressively obstinate with his parents and the
doctor when they remonstrate him." Obsessing about blood-
sugar levels (at any age) increases this anxiety. If your child's
levels are consistently out-of-whack, it may mean you have
to revamp her control regimen. Speak to your doctor.

As your child gets a little older (or if she's diagnosed
between ages eight and twelve, as many Type-I diabetics
are), she can start understanding that her diabetes makes her
different from her peers — and she may feel as if she has to
be super-perfect in every other area to compensate. Let's face
it: Children today are under a great deal of pressure to
"perform" from day one, whether they're 100 percent
healthy or chronically ill. As one mother we interviewed
pointed out, "No matter how sick your child is, you want her
to reach her full potential." This is fine — and parental en-

couragement is part of what motivates children to excellence — but be careful not to push your child to feel that because she has diabetes she has to be twice as good as her peers in everything else. This is not just unfair and unrealistic, it may make her feel she's being punished for diabetes, which in turn creates the false belief that it must, somehow, be her fault that she has it in the first place.

At ages eight through twelve, the ability to understand that diabetes is a medical condition, not a punishment, will increase dramatically. As Paula Liguori notes "The eight-year-olds are great, because they want to prove how much they can do, and how brave they are." Patti Keenan, whose son was diagnosed at age five, says the hardest challenge for her right now is having a six-year-old be so independent. "Diabetic children grow up so fast," she says, "It's important to let them be children and do what other kids do — as long as it doesn't hurt their diabetes."

"You must learn to provide supervision while giving your child responsibility to learn self-care and control," another mother from the Midwest told us. "Allow your child to participate to the full extent of his ability."

Diabetic children often miss out on the spontaneity that is usually the hallmark of childhood. They inherit a huge responsibility at the time of diagnosis, and often become "mini-adults" immediately.

"The diabetes becomes an arena for them to show off," says Paula Liguori about the eight-year-olds she works with. "If they're showing off by testing their blood properly and getting interested in giving their own shots, that's terrific."

Let it *be* terrific . . . and try not to resent your child's growing self-determination. It's not a rejection at all, but an acceptance — an acceptance of responsibility, say the doctors, and an acceptance of the reality that until a cure for diabetes is found, each diabetic must control his own disease.

Besides, all this self-determination may just fly out the window when your child hits the teenage years. "The problem with teenagers," says Paula Liguori, "is that one day they feel like being grown-up — and they'll do everything they're supposed to — and the next day they're totally irresponsible. That's why it's important not to throw the responsibility for diabetes control into your child's lap, even when it looks like he should be able to handle all the testing and shots on his own."

It's ironic. The older your child gets, the more important it is for her to control her blood sugar. But unfortunately, as your child passes through the teen years, she probably will adhere less to her regimen.

Around their twelfth birthdays, even the nicest kids can turn into teenage monsters. Rebellion is a normal part of being a teenager, but the teenager with diabetes has a very real and powerful weapon: When he or she wants to strike back at parents or siblings — or at the world — a teen with diabetes might stop taking shots on time, or start eating foods that are bad for her.

Because young people have a sense of immortality, they don't accept the fact that they're jeopardizing their own health this way; they just know that they're driving their parents crazy, which is exactly the desired effect!

If your teen is using diabetes as a weapon against you, don't make diabetes a battleground; in a battle, one side has to "win" — and if your child sees following her health regime as "losing" the battle, she will fight even harder to prove that she's the boss — and will take even less consistent care of herself.

Separating from one's parents is an important part of a

teenager's development, and feeling they need to depend on Mom and Dad because of the diabetes just makes kids resent the disease (and sometimes their parents) a little bit more. Therefore, we have found it tremendously important for Casey to have someone outside the family—someone she doesn't have to share with her sisters or even with us—to talk to, complain to, and gripe to.

We're tremendously pleased with the psychologist she has been seeing, and recommend that parents of all teenagers with diabetes seek out *someone*—be it a therapist, a physician, or even a friend of the family—that your teenager can talk to. Even the best therapist can't make the teenage years smooth for your child (or for any child). But a trained professional or sensitive advisor can help your teen learn how to express his or her individuality and frustrations in ways that are not damaging in the long run. Ages thirteen through eighteen are the hardest time for a young person with diabetes—just as they're the hardest years for *any* child (and their parents!). But the teen years can be especially tough on the families of diabetics because, as nurse-practitioner Penny Buschman explains, "Illness and treatment provide a whole other forum for parents and children to wage their battles in. A pre-adolescent or adolescent will act out with their disease, just as they act out in other areas. What happens when an adolescent goes to a party? She knows she's not supposed to have Coca-Cola, but half the adolescent diabetics I see do binge occasionally. Often, they'll leave the candy wrappers lying around to show their parents that they've been eating them." Some teenagers act out with their insulin regimes. Part of this comes from "testing" the adults, from wanting to see if the grownups really know what they're talking about when they warn about the consequences of missing a shot. "It's hard enough for families to survive the teen years," notes Buschman, "but when concern of physical danger exists, there's even more pressure."

When they're under pressure, teenagers (*all* teenagers!) are notorious for storming into their rooms, slamming doors, and refusing to talk to anyone for days. But it is critical that you and your child keep the lines of communications open, and that you can talk to your child about the peer pressures that can make the teen years so trying for every teenager — and so fraught with challenges for those with diabetes. All the things that regular parents warn their teenagers about are especially dangerous for your child, so it's important that you give all the "standard-issue lectures" in a way that will make your child listen. Drinking to excess or abusing drugs is foolish for everyone, but especially for a teenager who may, if drunk or high, forget to take a shot or test his blood. Besides, alcohol turns rapidly into sugar, which is very harmful to the diabetic. Because pot sets off the munchies while lowering reasoning ability, smoking is a bad idea for people who need to watch their diets and make clear-headed choices about how much to eat and when.

Even a beer or two can be harmful to the diabetic teenager for a less obvious reason. A child with liquor on his breath is likely to be assumed drunk by the police, even if he's had just a few sips. Imagine this scenario: Your teenager has half a glass or so of beer at a party, and, still sober, starts driving home. His blood sugar starts to dip, and he weaves on the road, alerting a cop to pull him over. The policeman, smelling the beer and noting that the teen can't walk a straight line, takes him down to the station to question him — or maybe just to shake him up a little. The time your child spends at the police station without food can contribute to a serious insulin reaction.

If your teenager won't listen to *you* when you talk about these issues, find an adult figure who *isn't* a parent or teacher that she *will* talk to. An aunt or uncle, or a close friend of yours can serve as a sounding board for your child's concerns about things she might not want to discuss with you. Sure, we all want to think that our kids are being 100 percent honest with us 100 percent of the time, but were you that honest with your parents? Do you know anyone who was? Kids need secrets from their parents. It's part of the natural separation process. But with diabetic children, whose "secrets" might have long-term effects on their health, it is important that someone, somewhere, is getting the whole picture of your child's life. If your physician can be this sounding board, so much the better. She will know for sure whether your child's behavior is dangerous, and will have more practical advice about handling situations that arise.

The teen years are full of parent-child battles for every family, but when your child has diabetes, remember: before you pick a fight, choose your fights carefully. You and your diabetic child will undoubtedly be at loggerheads about aspects of her medical regime, and it's important for you to stand firm on those issues. But every kid needs a bit of wiggle room—room to try out different behavior and to annoy the daylights out of her parents. When your child has to contend with a string of thou shall's and thou shalt not's that are part of living with diabetes, that wiggle room becomes all the more precious—and all the more important to your child's growing sense of self.

For Casey, whose school has strict dress codes and behavior rules, finding an area of rebellion was a challenge. But like most teens, she rose to that challenge and figured out just how to get our goat without facing school expulsion or diabetic complications: She chose to draw the battle lines around her hairdo and we decided that it was in the whole family's best interest not to cross — or even threaten — those lines.

Is peroxide-blonde with dark roots our fantasy hairstyle for our teenage daughter? Not at all — though we suppose it's better than electric blue hair or a shaved head. But asserting her independence in this way affects Casey no longer than it will take her hair to return to her natural honey-blonde color. Skipping shots or drinking alcohol, on the other hand, could leave her — or any diabetic child — with consequences that last into and all through their adulthood. So we've kept the hair issue a *non*issue, and remind ourselves daily that a "bad hair year" is better than a bad hypoglycemic reaction.

You don't have to love your child's hairdo — or that fourth hole in her earlobe or the grunge look. But when it comes to your child's looks, it's often better to look the other way. Save the insistence and parental rank-pulling for things like diabetic self-care and good exercise habits — that will affect your child in the long run.

"Pay attention to the special needs of adolescents," advised Lawrence Kutner in his "Parent & Child" column on chronically ill children. "Children this age are struggling to gain their independence from their parents. One way they can do this is by making more of their own choices, so that they do not have to focus on their health care as a point of rebellion."

To keep the natural teenage rebellion within nondestructive boundaries, Dr. Ginsberg suggests that you "give in on the messy room, on the haircut. But make sure your teenager knows that taking her insulin shot is non-negotiable. Sometimes we even make deals with our patients," she told us. "A teenager will say, 'If my father lets me pierce my ear, I'll take my shots.' We encourage the parents to go along with this. After all, if the kid decides he doesn't like the hole ten years down the line, he can let it close up, but if he does damage to his nervous system, it's irreparable."

So give your child some leeway on the loud music, the two-different-color socks. Before you get obsessed with what diabetes is doing to your child's taste, judgment, or sartorial sense, remember that the punk-rocker look (or the bookishness or the affected Scottish accent) may have nothing whatsoever to do with your child's diabetes at all. As Lawrence Kutner wrote, "It's not unusual for parents to ascribe totally unrelated problems to a chronic illness. By focusing on their child's weaknesses rather than strengths, they may unconsciously be teaching those children to feel helpless and not in control." Feeling in control is a big part of what helps diabetic children and adolescents remain hopeful and productive despite the severity of the illness.

That's why, whenever it's medically possible, you should try and let your *child's* feelings be your guide. We finally stopped trying to get Casey to play with other diabetic children, despite all the studies that show that diabetic kids who attend special camps have a great time and increase their self-esteem and diabetes control. She simply doesn't want to hang around with other diabetic children.

As Casey explained in chapter one of this book, she doesn't want to associate with people who are diabetic, because then other people will look at her like she's different, or "sickly." Whatever the reason, we've come to realize that since there are so many areas of dealing with her diabetes that are, as Dr. Ginsberg puts it, "non-negotiable" it's a good idea to let Casey call the shots (no pun intended) about some of the things—like choosing her own friends—that don't adversely affect her health.

Try to give *your* child some room, too. If she wants some privacy when it comes to her diabetes, try your best to grant it. If, on the other hand, she feels comfortable about testing her glucose in a room full of people, don't encourage her to leave the room. A friend who works with childhood cancer patients tells a wonderfully illustrative story. Each summer, when the children arrive for the cancer camp where she volunteers, their heads are covered by wigs—but as soon as they're out of the parking lot and their parents can't see them, the children whip off their head coverings. They are perfectly comfortable—especially around each other—with their condition. It's their parents who are self-conscious. Diabetic children, too, are often less self-conscious than parents, and sometimes (as seems to be the case with Casey) they are a bit *more* reserved about sharing the details of their disease. Let your child decide what amount of exposure (both in terms of routine procedures in public and in public knowledge of her problem) makes her comfortable, and try to let her work out on her own how she feels most comfortable coping with "being different."

Remember that some of your child's "differences" will actually serve her well. Diabetic children are usually more mature, self-confident, and self-reliant than their peers. Despite all our talk about spiked hairdos and twenty-three earrings, many children with diabetes channel their feelings of "differentness" into areas of excellence. Their leadership qualities make diabetic children popular, and their determination makes them successful. The challenges they face during their youth and adolescence often strengthen children with diabetes into adults who can handle life's curve balls and make themselves and their parents proud.

7

Your Diabetic Child at School and at Play

With all the things we parents of kids with diabetes have to worry about, it's always refreshing to hear some *good* news: Studies show no difference in the academic achievement of diabetic children and their healthy peers. Lots of kids with diabetes make it to—and through—the finest colleges and professional schools, and the legions of successful adults who have had diabetes since childhood prove that diabetes need not limit your child's accomplishments.

But while your child's diabetes probably won't affect her school performance in the long run, don't be too alarmed if her grades go down a bit at first. She might be distracted by the stress of diagnosis, and until her sugar levels are really closely controlled, she may have occasional problems concentrating.

The most common reason for academic problems among newly diagnosed diabetics is the simplest: It can take quite a bit of time and extra work to make up on a few weeks' missed classes. Try to keep these catch-up struggles in check over the long haul, and try to keep your child in school as much as possible.

If the doctor *has* ordered your child to stay at home for a certain period of time, let the teachers and principals know up front what the expected duration of the absence will be. In many school districts, a teacher is available for hospital tutoring. In an article on "Potential Problems for Chronically Ill Children in Schools" in the *Peabody Journal of Education,* the authors wrote, "In most states, children absent for more than two weeks receive homebound or hospital instruction under the aegis of the special-education department. This required waiting time does not help the child with frequent intermittent absences to keep current on academics. For this child, the potential to develop school phobia is thought to be greater."

Plan ahead for missed days to minimize the "school phobia" caused by being behind on assignments. Who will bring your child's assignments home? Who will let her copy notes? Knowing that she will be able to catch up to her classmates will help put your child at ease both during her initial hospitalization and during any subsequent absences.

Even if your child needs a little extra help outside school, work with teachers to see that she's treated as "normally" as possible *in* school. The more typically you can treat a child, the better she feels about herself. The better a child feels about herself, the better she will do in school, and in life.

To make your child's school days healthier and less stressful, meet with her teachers and work *with* them on your child's behalf. If your child is still in elementary school, it's also helpful if you can spend a few days trouble-shooting while she makes the transition from the hospital or clinic to the playground and the classroom.

The first day Casey went back to school, we gave a little demonstration to her class. We showed them what a syringe looks like, and Casey got up in front of the class and tested her blood. There's no question that the blood and needles were initially very upsetting for some of Casey's classmates; they were only in third grade. But we think our frankness about diabetes eliminated any mystery — and potential gossip — and her classmates soon got as used to Casey's routine as she is.

Accompanying your child to school will not only help you ease her transition socially, but will give you the chance to get teachers up to speed on your child's new routine and alert them to the danger signs to look for, and will allow you to make sure there is *someone* supervising your child. A while back, a mother called Sale for some advice on how to handle the following situation: Her three-year-old son had recently been diagnosed, and had just gone back to nursery school. Both the parents work full time, so they had made a special effort to explain to the teachers as best they could what their son could and couldn't eat and what he could and couldn't do. But we all know how tough it is to supervise a three-year-old boy, especially in a class of thirty-three children. So the child was frequently going low and having hypoglycemic emergencies. Other times, he was eating sweets that other kids brought, and he was going high. Sale suggested that they check the child's blood sugar more often and give the teacher a specific list of which snacks should be given at which blood-sugar levels. That seemed to help the family cope and now they're as convinced as we are that constant dialogue with school personnel is vital.

If you can accompany your child to school for a few days, try to do so. By the time Casey was discharged from the hospital she had just two weeks left of school before summer vacation, so Sale went with her every day. You may not want to tag along for two full weeks, but it is a good idea to take a couple of days off to accompany a young child to school on her first few days after diagnosis. In addition to having a new regimen to adapt to, she will probably experience some sugar-level fluctuations when the insulin doses your doctor prescribed in the calm of a hospital are subjected to the running and jumping of elementary school.

While you will not have to accompany a teenager to school at all once you and he have explained diabetes to the teachers, do make sure you all sit down and clarify who's responsible for each aspect of care. This helps eliminate the snafus that can occur when each person thinks someone else is carrying the insulin, and will avoid the power struggles that can result when a teenager starts pitting school personnel against parents.

Whatever your child's age, you should be sure to investigate the system her school has put in place. Does it provide your child with both enough supervision to minimize the risk of high- and low-sugar episodes and enough freedom to be a "regular kid"?

Find out if the school has an official policy about children with chronic illnesses, and how those policies affect your child. Some schools, for example, will not let a child carry her own syringes, partly out of misguided fear that other children will use them for drugs and partly because they're worried that your child might lose her needles. Push for your child's right to have her own equipment, and provide a clearly labeled spare for the classroom and another for the nurse's office. You may want to follow the lead of a family we interviewed, who donated a glucose monitor to the school.

When working—or negotiating—with your child's

school, bear in mind that while most schools do genuinely want to provide your child with a healthful, supportive environment, over 50 percent of the schools in this country have no school nurse. This shortage usually leaves teachers with no knowledge of diabetes to care for your child.

Therefore, Shirley Swope, parent advisor at the PEAK Parent Information Center in Colorado Springs, suggests that your first approach should be to talk to the teachers directly. After all, she says, most of them went into education because they genuinely like children. Explain your child's illness to them, and make sure they understand the steps your child has to take to stay healthy.

Most of the time this works, but occasionally, because of their own fear of the unknown and stress levels, teachers are less than cooperative. "When Mark was first diagnosed," a mother told us, "his second-grade teacher was totally insensitive to his condition. She told me she didn't know why this kind of thing was happening to *her*."

Try to work out this kind of problem directly with the teacher if you can. Usually, understanding diabetes a little better helps people feel more at ease about supervising a diabetic child. If your child's teacher is really making life difficult for you and your child, talk to the school's special education director. He or she is in charge of seeing that every child gets the education she deserves and needs regardless of "disability."

"Know that you can keep going up the ladder if you have trouble," says Judy Haley, "but don't start asking for help from a position of anger. Start with smiling confidence, knowing that the school can't wait to accommodate your needs, and they're more likely to do so!"

Indeed, most parents find that schools *do* cooperate: "My

daughter just started high school," one mother told us, delightedly. "We met with the school nurse, who sent letters to all her teachers. We were amazed to learn that they keep a blood glucose meter and strips at school, even though there are only a handful of diabetics in the school."

Even in schools that are less well equipped, you can help ensure your child's good health if you are willing to meet them halfway—or sometimes 75 percent of the way. "I've always had good cooperation with the schools," says Susan Briston, "but I have been a pushy mother, too. For example, my daughter's kindergarten teacher announced a field trip in the first week of school with no adult helpers! I said 'I'm coming too,' and it turned out she needed me just to help with the other children, besides caring for my own child."

If either you or your spouse is a full-time at-home parent, you may want to think about volunteering at your child's school. With state and local budget cuts, schools need all the extra hands they can get. The more visible you are, the more likely you are to be told about "minor" problems that the teachers might not communicate if they had to call you or arrange a special conference.

Even if you *are* around your child's school often, the best way to deal with problems is to *prevent* them. And the best way to do *that,* of course, is with teamwork and good communication. "The better partnership parents can have with their child's school," says Shirley Swope, "the better education the child receives. If your child has a serious illness like diabetes, dealing with problems at school can be one more stress—another stress that parents don't cope with as well as they would in another, calmer, time in their lives. Often, the schools lose sight of the fact that parents are under so much stress with the child's illness. They can't understand why the parents are having such a tough time dealing with what appears to the school to be a minor problem."

Remember, in the midst of any stress that crops up, that you accomplish your goals best if you can communicate with your child's teachers in a way that lets them know you trust them and respect them. Be sure you're not insulting or condescending when you explain symptoms and procedures. After your child returns from the hospital and then again at the beginning of every school year, meet with your child's teachers, principals, and the school nurse.

The Juvenile Diabetes Foundation publishes a brochure, called *A Child with Diabetes Is in Your Care,* that your child's teachers and school administrators may find helpful. It explains the disease and lets them know what to do if your child has either a high-sugar or a low-sugar reaction.

Don't forget a copy of the brochure (and some in-person advice) for the gym teacher. Activity is much more likely to set off an insulin reaction than spelling class is. There is absolutely no reason a diabetic child can't participate fully in sports. Just make sure you take extra activity into account when planning meals and snacks.

Besides educating your child's regular teachers, make sure there are provisions for alerting substitutes to your child's conditions and needs. Leave extra copies of JDF's brochure for teachers with your child's principal or whoever is in charge of coordinating substitute-teacher check-in.

Making sure all the right people are informed makes sense legally, too. If there's a negligence-caused accident at school and you decide to sue, the school will not be held liable if they were not provided with all the appropriate information. We don't know of any cases where this has been necessary, though. Just make sure all the teachers know how to use the "tools of the trade." Show them how your child's glucose monitor is used, and how to smear honey on her gums if she's having a reaction and can't swallow food. Also, make sure each educator responsible for your child knows what to do—and whom to call—in an emergency.

Tell the school bus driver about your child's diabetes, and give him emergency supplies. A fifteen-minute bus ride home can turn into an all-afternoon ordeal if the bus breaks down and has to wait for repairs or an alternate vehicle. When this happened to Casey once, we were glad she was prepared.

Be sure to tell your child's teacher how diabetes might affect his concentration or behavior. It's amazing how many children are labeled behavior problems because their teachers are ignoring signs that there's a sugar problem. If you suspect this has already tarnished your child's school records, insist on seeing her files and include notations as you see fit. Under the family rights and privacy act, parents of a student under eighteen years of age must be permitted to inspect and review all records maintained by the school district. If parents feel that some information in the record is inaccurate or misleading, they may place in the records a statement commenting on or disagreeing with the information. Your school's guidance counselor or school psychologist can help you and your child with these issues, and is also an excellent resource if your child needs someone to speak to about her feelings or concerns.

Make sure teachers have quick-acting sugar, like orange juice in those shelf-stable cartons or some candy, handy for emergencies. To *avoid* low blood sugars, make sure the teacher knows that your child can never miss his scheduled eating times. "No snack" is as common a punishment in

schools as "no dessert" is in many homes. But for the diabetic, either of these measures can be disruptive at mini-
mum, and in some cases even dangerous. Casey has always
been allowed to leave the classroom for her snack, but in
some schools, this is impossible, and the diabetic child must
eat her snack at her desk. In an article by Barbara Balik,
Broatch Haig, and Patricia Moynihan, the authors stress the
use of "low-noise" foods for snacks. Peanut butter sand-
wiches make less crunching noises than potato chips, and
besides being a more nutritious choice, they're quieter to eat
in the classroom.

Remember that the snacks you send from home are only
a part of what your child consumes each day at school.
Check the school food carefully to see that it's not only
balanced, but tasty enough that your child will actually eat
it. Her friends may skip the creamed chipped beef with no
ill effect, but a diabetic child cannot afford to miss lunch. If
the school cafeteria food is, in the kids' word, "gross," send
a bag lunch, or arrange for your child's food to be kept in the
school kitchen.

If your child *does* become ill in class because of a missed
meal or snack (or for any other reason) and needs to go to the
administrative or nurse's office, make sure the teacher
knows to send another student along. Hypoglycemic children often get confused, and your child might get lost or
even pass out if she's suffering from very low blood sugar.

Also make sure that in addition to understanding diabetes
itself, each of the adults responsible for your child in school
understands *your* expectations of how they should help you
manage the illness. Not all children are on the same regimen.
Make sure your child's teacher is responding to *your* child,
and not to a preconceived idea of what diabetes is and how

it should be treated. Many people who think they know about diabetes have only had experience with Type-II, which is treated quite differently.

It's a good idea to discuss with your child's teacher the level of privacy you and your child expect, too. Some children are self-conscious and don't want their problem mentioned in class. Others can't wait to bring their glucose monitors to show-and-tell.

While the law safeguards many aspects of your child's privacy, experts at the Connecticut Parent Advocacy Center suggest that you give doctors and educators some extra latitude in discussing your child's progress with one another. "Share the sources of information about your child's needs (pediatrician, specialist, therapist) and give permission for the school nurse to consult with these professionals if there are questions," they say. "Also, give permission for the school nurse to share relevant information with teachers who are working with your child." To retain as much privacy as possible, insist that this is done in person, in meetings between the teacher and the nurse, not in circulated memos that could be left lying around the teachers' desks where other students might read them.

Recently, Casey changed schools, to one with smaller classes. We find that when her teachers have more time to pay attention to her progress, she is less likely to fall behind in her studies due to low blood-sugar episodes. Regardless of your child's class size, make sure the teachers know how to recognize when your child needs some extra help or reinforcement.

Once you've explained diabetes and its ramifications to school personnel, it's a good idea for you and/or your child to spend some time clarifying things for her friends, too. Particularly if your child has been in the hospital, there are sure to be a lot of questions and fears flying around her classroom when she returns. "Is diabetes catching?" "Is Johnny going to die?" There were certainly a lot of questions going around with Casey's friends, and we're glad we cleared them up with our show-and-tell before they got out of hand or made Casey feel uncomfortable around her classmates.

Sure, we have heard of a few cases where children were "picked on" because of their diabetes, but like most biases and stigmas, a classmate's nasty reaction to your child's illness can usually be quelled with a healthy dose of information. Although Casey felt a bit self-conscious when she first demonstrated her procedures to her class, she agrees that in the long run, her openness has gone a long way to making her life at school and at play with her friends a lot easier.

Other parents have found the show-and-tell route helpful, too. Ellen Smith wrote us that "when Debbie returned to school after being diagnosed, I went with her one day and she did a demonstration with all her equipment and we talked to her class. It was amazing how curious and insightful fourth graders can be."

It's amazing, too, how helpful their *parents* can be once you've explained to them briefly what your child can and can't eat and what signs of a reaction they should look out for. "In the beginning," says Mrs. Smith, "there was one mother who was afraid to have Debbie play at her house. But that changed, and all is fine now. I talk to the parents before birthday parties and sleepovers, and everyone is wonderful about providing alternative treats for her."

"Our friends have been wonderful," says the mother of a

young boy. "I always check out the menu at parties prior to the date. I do allow my son to eat some treats within reason. After all, he is a child, and he does know his limits."

"I found the parents of my son's friends to be very helpful and willing to discuss and learn about Sean's diet and care while under their supervision," says another mother.

One parent advised that "teachers can send suggestions for healthy snacks for treats and parties at school to all parents without mentioning the child who has diabetes. Most parents are happy to have less junk food around even if their kids *don't* have diabetes." We wish Casey's school would implement this! We'd love to see our other daughters benefit from some nutrition awareness, too.

Of course, the only thing kids like more than birthday parties is, you guessed it, summer vacation, and diabetic children are no different. What *does* differ is the extra attention you'll have to pay to sugar levels when your child's on the less predictable schedule that comes along with those lazy, hazy, crazy days of summer.

After she was released from the hospital, and just when we got Casey adjusted to school, the term was over and her day-to-day activities changed again. You, too, will probably have to fine-tune your child's diet, exercise, and insulin regime at different times of the year. Kids are a lot more active on vacation, which can make the summer and Christmas time a little more challenging.

A little advance planning can go a long way toward making vacation travel less stressful and healthier for everyone. In an article in the *New York Times* in the summer of 1991, health writer Jane Brody made the following suggestions for traveling with diabetes:

• If you're traveling, be sure to put enough medical supplies in your carry-on bag to last the entire trip plus one extra week. Make sure to keep the syringes in their original package and carry your insulin prescription. Needles aren't the easiest thing to get through airport security, as you might imagine. Some parents carry a physician's letter describing their child's condition and medical needs as extra backup.

• If you are flying to your destination, take plenty of snacks on the plane to account for the fact that these days more planes leave late than on time. If your plane sits on the ground an extra six hours, you may be stuck with no food service on the plane and no way to get off and buy anything.

• If you're flying across time zones, you'll have to adjust your child's insulin schedule to match new mealtimes. Talk to your doctor about the best way to do this without jolting your child's system.

• Once you get where you're going, remember that sunburns that peel heal more slowly for diabetics, and that walking on the beach barefoot can lead to little cuts. Sunscreen and flip-flops will help you avoid these problems.

• Finally, because diabetics have to be especially careful about systemic infections, be careful about where you let your child drink the water. Note that in places where you shouldn't drink the water, you shouldn't eat washed vegetables or unpeeled fruits, or drink beverages with ice cubes, either.

If your child has always spent summer vacation at camp, she can continue to do so. Many "regular" sleep-away and day camps will accept diabetic children, and there are many others specifically for kids with diabetes. Although we have never sent Casey to a special camp because she has shied away from playing with other kids with diabetes, everyone we know who *has* attended diabetes camp has had a ball, and gained not only new friends but better control, a better understanding of their diabetes, and a healthy boost to their self-esteem.

"Mark was asked to be a counselor at a diabetes camp because of the great attitude and self-esteem he had developed," one proud mother told us. Others said that the supportive environment of diabetes camp had helped their child adjust to the illness and return to school more relaxed and ready to learn.

Your child may feel more comfortable with the friends she makes in diabetes camp or, like Casey, may shy away from other kids with diabetes. Either way, your diabetic child needs what we all do: friends who care; friends who are there. If you teach your child to use her diabetes as an inspiration rather than an excuse, and to share information and feelings with her friends, there is absolutely no reason she can't enjoy that kind of close relationship with her schoolmates, neighborhood friends, and even, with a little luck, her family!

8

Diabetes and Your Family

There's no question that Casey's diabetes has affected our family in a very profound way. The NASA-like precision of scheduling, the daily stress of worrying about our daughter's health, and the extra time and attention we give Casey have affected each of us — and the way we relate to one another.

Any parent with more than one child must try to balance the attention she gives each. When that balance is thrown off by one child's special needs, the other children are likely to feel jealous. All marriages need time — and time without the kids — to keep them healthy. When an ill child absorbs a great deal of that time, partners have to work doubly hard to keep themselves and their relationship strong. Over the past few years we have grappled with all of these issues, learning along the way and trying to correct the inevitable mistakes that we, like parents of *any* children, might make.

Despite all the stresses, we feel that in many ways, Casey's diabetes has taught us all, as a family, a great deal about each other and about working together. We've had to learn to communicate more effectively, to handle stress and family conflicts, and not to sweat the small stuff. We've also had to be careful about making sure that we control Casey's diabetes — and not the other way around.

The better everyone in your family understands diabetes — and each other — the better you will all be able to adjust to your child's condition. If you are having family problems because of the changes your child's diabetes has made in your life, go speak to someone together.

"All families are affected to some extent when diabetes is diagnosed," says Dr. Ginsberg. "So help at the beginning may be important for the whole family. Later on, your teenager may want to go talk to someone herself."

The counselor you see right after your child's diagnosis need not be a child psychologist, says Dr. Maryann Feldstein, R.N., C.E., Ed.D., a psychotherapist in New York City "because there is not necessarily something amiss with the child, per se. Instead, ask your physician to recommend a counselor who understands how families work and how a child's diabetes can affect that functioning. In some families, for instance, diabetes distracts family members from other conflicts. If a child senses a fight brewing between mother and father, she may have a diabetic crisis, because her subconscious wishes to divert their attention."

Of course, the flip side to *masking* family problems with the diabetes is unfairly blaming conflicts on the disease. In *Meeting the Challenge of Disability,* authors Lori A. Goldfarb, Mary Jane Brotherson, Jean Ann Summers, and Ann P. Turnbull point out that "the tendency to attribute the cause of family problems to a member's illness or disability can be a dangerous lure and trap for families. . . . Furthermore, it can distract from the true source of a problem and, thus, can camouflage a number of useful solutions."

Even in the healthiest of families, diabetes can intensify

any conflicts that may have been lying dormant before a child's diagnosis. Like any stress, a child's diabetes can make strong families stronger and weak families weaker. "Before the stress [of a chronic illness]" writes Dr. T. Berry Brazelton in his book, *Families: Crisis and Caring* (Ballantine, 1989), "everything may have looked and felt fine — on the surface. It is only under stress that we become aware of underlying rivalries, fears, weak links in family attachments. For each member of a family, this is a period of doubt and confusion. Can I muster enough energy to meet the new demands? Can we as a family band together to offer each other the strength we will need? Despite the pain and discomfort of such a period, a kind of emotional adrenaline courses through the family and this very sense of disorganization makes room for growth and change."

The emotional adrenaline is at its peak soon after families learn about a member's diabetes. To channel that heightened energy in a positive way and minimize the fear and anxiety that can overtake the family, be sure to share as much information as you can with your non-diabetic children right from the beginning. Changes in the family affect children in a profound way, and even the youngest children will sense that something is wrong. The more information you can share with them — both about what's happening to their sibling and about ways family life might change — the more easily they'll adjust to their sibling's illness and the changes it brings to the family.

Younger children are especially likely to be frightened when a sibling is ill. They're likely to be wondering whether their sister is going to die, and scared, too, that they might catch the disease. Be sure to explain diabetes to the whole family in terms appropriate to each member's age. Make sure everyone understands that while there may be an increased likelihood of their developing diabetes if it runs in the family, the chance is still very small (only 5 to 8 percent, according to Dr. Ginsberg). Your doctor, diabetes educator, or social worker can help you develop an explanation that is honest and accurate without being frightening or overladen with medical jargon.

Because well-controlled diabetes has few visible symptoms, young children often can't understand what all the fuss is about if their diabetic brother or sister looks and acts fine after leaving the hospital. Therefore, it's especially important to explain carefully that your child's illness is only serious if it's *not* treated properly, and that all the attention you're lavishing on the child is necessary to prevent long-term complications.

"There's a lot of rage among siblings of chronically ill children, and a lot of rivalry is added," says Penny Buschman, R.N., C.E., an Assistant Professor at Columbia University School of Nursing. "Siblings may think they caused the illness or may worry that they're next in line to catch it. It's important to encourage the family to talk about this, and it's important to make sure from the beginning that siblings understand what goes on in the hospital or the clinic, so they know that all the time their sick brother or sister is getting isn't 'special' time, and so they don't become resentful."

Even when you explain (and explain, and explain) to your non-diabetic children why there's an inequity in the attention you're doling out, they're likely to feel slighted. "My older daughter is lacking the attention she should have," said one mother we interviewed. "She feels her sister is treated better than she is."

When a diabetic sibling is cornering the market on mom

and dad's time, the *non*-diabetic siblings often act out to get the attention they feel is being denied to them. "The imbalance sets up a conflict," explains Dr. Maryann Feldstein. "The healthy children may resent all the attention (and, often, presents) that their diabetic sibling gets and may start acting up at school. Face it," says Dr. Feldstein. "Kids get more attention when they're bad than when they're good."

If you start noticing behavior problems in your non-diabetic children, do not just ignore them and hope they'll go away over time (the problems *or* the kids!). Bottled-up feelings can build over the long run and explode suddenly, when you least expect it and are least prepared to handle a family crisis. Remember that as distressing as your kid's acting-out may be, it actually may be healthier than the other common reaction to anger against an ill sibling or the parents, which is to hold it in and seethe. At least the acting out alerts parents that a problem exists and gives them the opportunity to nip it in the bud.

"The best way to do that," says Dr. Feldstein, "is to be sure to give each child special time alone with each of you. Use that time to focus on activities that make each child feel different and special."

Dr. Feldstein also suggests that you make sure to be vocally appreciative when your non-diabetic children do something helpful to their diabetic brother or sister. This not only encourages helpfulness, she says, "but reassures your child that despite all the attention you've been paying to doctors, hospitals, and illnesses, you are still aware of how important his or her contributions to the family are."

Siblings can help you recognize—and avert—an impending diabetic crisis if you teach them the signs to watch for. If your kids share a room, let siblings know that lots of

tossing and turning can be a sign of a nighttime hypoglycemia reaction. Teach them how to handle a daytime insulin
shock, as well. But don't overburden them with responsibility for their sibling's care. Most diabetics hate feeling like
somebody's watching over their shoulder, and your child
may come to resent her sister's watchful eye.

So might the "watcher." Be careful not to limit your praise
to diabetes-related helpfulness. "Saying 'Isn't he wonderful!'
each time your healthy child helps his diabetic brother sets
up a cycle in which the healthy child feels that the caretaker
role is what assures his position in the family," says Dr.
Feldstein.

In fact, she says, "It's amazing how many people in the
helping professions grew up with sick siblings. They grow
up seeing their role as caretakers, and that carries over into
their professional choices." There are better ways to get your
non-diabetic daughter to be a doctor. Try buying her a chem-
istry set! "She cares for her sister like a nurse when I'm not
around," one mother we interviewed said of her non-diabetic child. "Sometimes, it worries me."

"Often," says Feldstein, "the healthy children feel guilty,
either for being healthy while their sibling is suffering the
indignities of shots and special diets, or sometimes, in
younger children, in thinking they somehow caused the
disease. As irrational as that guilt is, it often continues
through to adulthood."

In understanding your non-diabetic children's response
to their sibling's diabetes, be mindful of the fact that in
families with a chronically ill child, the healthy children
often feel badly that they *are* healthy while a much-loved
brother or sister is subjected to daily shots and pinpricks. "I
feel my younger daughter has guilt about being 'the healthy

child'," a mother told us. "I never realized this until she wrote her college essay on her sister." You must be sensitive to the pain, guilt, and inequities that can arise when one child in the family has diabetes, and pay careful attention to what your non-diabetic children are thinking and feeling.

Penny Buschman notes that parents often ignore their healthy children's concerns because having a sick child can make all other problems pale. "So, if your daughter's diabetes rates a 10 on the scale of 1 to 10, your other child's failed math test is only a two," she says. "It's important to recognize that to *her* it's a 10. Don't say, 'How can you complain about that when your sister has worse problems?' Each child's problems are important to him."

Ironically, some parents feel like they're "punishing" their healthy children by converting the whole family to the diabetic's diet. Nothing could be further from the truth. The diabetic's diet is healthful, and since your non-diabetic children can eat junk food at birthday parties and at friends' houses, eliminating the temptations at home serves everyone's best interests. Still, non-diabetic children often resent having to do without sweets at home simply because it's too tempting for the diabetic child to have goodies around the house. Many complain about having to follow the diabetic child's rigid schedule, when they'd rather eat on the fly.

Some of the guilt and resentment siblings feel is unavoidable, but there are things you can do to minimize them. There is a difference between saying, "Please be quiet, your brother isn't feeling well today," and saying "How can you make noise when your brother is sleeping?" Note that distinction, and don't intervene every time a normal, brotherly squabble breaks out. Often, when healthy children "pick on" a diabetic sibling in normal ways, they're told they have to stop.

(Of course in our house, the younger two are so busy being picked *on* by their older sister that they have little time left to antagonize Casey.) Remember that a little yelling, screaming, and tattletaling, not to mention a few flailing fists and stuck-out tongues, are all part of the normal family experience. Trying to shield your diabetic child from this standard part of growing up is counterproductive, both to her and to your other children's feelings of normalcy.

Maintaining that normalcy can be tricky, but it has its payoffs. Children who grow up around someone who needs care often come to understand the value of patience and compassion. "My daughter's illness has actually been good for my other children," one mother told us. "I feel my family is more sensitive to the health needs of other people, and more accepting of people's differences. But let me tell you, this didn't happen by osmosis. I spent a lot of time and a lot of hard work to achieve that. I taught my boys how they could help their sister, and I didn't tolerate any insensitivity, nor do I tolerate her disrespect for them. In fact, when my daughter complains about her brothers like all girls do, I remind her of all the ways they've helped her."

While you're focusing on how one child's diabetes affects your other kids, don't forget to spend some time thinking about whether, and how, the illness is affecting your marriage. No matter how strong your relationship with your spouse is, finding out your child has a serious illness can add a tremendous strain. Fear and anxiety take their toll, and the sheer number of hours you have to spend concentrating on and dealing with the everyday aspects of your child's treatment makes it difficult to spend as much time alone with your partner as you might like.

Like other relationships within the family, most strong

marriages can withstand the pressures of raising a diabetic child — *if* you're aware of potential problems so that you can fix them early on, before they escalate.

In his book, *Families: Crisis and Caring,* Dr. T. Berry Brazelton notes that "Detachment from the illness or from the child can occur in overwhelmed parents. They may not show up to stand by the sick child. They watch television in the child's room rather than paying attention to the child. Sometimes, it seems too much for parents to face pain in their own child and in the other children in the hospital." If your spouse doesn't seem to be paying enough attention to your diabetic child — or to you — this may be why. Try to talk these feelings over and let your spouse know how much you need him or her. Often, pulling away is a result of feeling helpless or guilty.

"The guilt over the child's diabetes can affect the parents' relationship too," says Dr. Feldstein. "One partner may secretly (or openly) blame the other for the illness, and may lash out with statements like "People on your side of the family have diabetes." Remember that while diabetes is a genetically-linked disease, it's not something we *give* our children — and it's certainly not something we can rationally fault ourselves or each other for.

Problems also can arise if one parent gets overinvolved, and develops an unhealthy attachment to the child that excludes the spouse. "Taking care of a young diabetic child can be a full-time affair," says Dr. Feldstein. "It's all too easy to get so wrapped up in keeping your child healthy that you forget that keeping marriages healthy also takes work."

A good marriage takes not only work but a fair division of labor. Caring for a diabetic child is a huge task for two parents. When it falls on the shoulders of one alone, resentment is bound to creep up. If you are divorced, decide who is responsible for which aspects of managing your child's interests. Look out for hidden burdens. You may decide to split medical costs 50/50, but if one of you gets stuck handling all the forms he or she might become resentful.

If one parent decides to stop working to take care of the sick child (it's usually the mother), she's likely to feel resentful about thwarted career goals. But sometimes, the family changes brought on by diabetes are happy surprises. "After Brandon was diagnosed, I quit my job to become a full-time mom," Sandra Gandy says. "I find that I love having the opportunity to spend more time with my children, volunteering at my daughter's school, and other things, despite the negative financial effects of not working anymore."

Try to keep your eyes open, though, to the possibility that if you or your spouse stop working or cut back on hours, the working partner may feel stressed-out by now having to be the sole bread winner. On the flip side, a mother who has made a careful decision to stay at home, but who now has to go to work to help pay for medical expenses, may feel overwhelmed.

To ease the strain and keep your marriage as healthy as possible, be sure to schedule time to be alone with your spouse. Don't let the fear of leaving your child with a babysitter keep you home, either. If you have a regular sitter, you can teach her about your child's diabetes the same way you teach grandparents and teachers. If you'd be more comfortable with someone who's already a diabetes expert, call your local chapter of JDF or ADA and find out if there are any local diabetic teenagers who want to earn some extra money from time to time by babysitting, or see if you can find a retired nurse.

It's a good idea to spend some of your time alone discussing your child's illness with your spouse, sharing not only emotions, but information, and working toward seeing any problems that arise the same way. In most families it's the mother who's responsible for taking the child to the doctor (or, if a baby-sitter is handling daytime appointments, the mother who gets the reports from her). Be sure you're letting your partner in on everything the professionals are telling you, and on everything significant you observe in your child. Both parents should go to the doctor's visits together, at least occasionally, so that the responsibility of absorbing and communicating information doesn't fall to one of you alone.

Be sure, too, to spend some time alone, focused on other things—like romance!

Susan Stautberg, co-author of *Managing It All* (MasterMedia), suggests the following strategies for couples who are having trouble making time for each other:

- Get up early and talk in bed.
- Exercise together first thing in the morning.
- If you work close to each other, meet for lunch.
- Take one or two "sick days" a year and play hookey together.

Juggling all the responsibilities of working (inside or outside the home), raising children, and worrying about diabetes control can sap some of your time and energy. Don't ignore that possibility. If you make a special effort to take time for each other (as well as for yourself, all alone—even if it means locking yourself in the bathroom with a good book!) the daily stresses are less likely to take their toll over time.

And if you look at diabetes not as an obstacle to family happiness but as a catalyst for greater closeness, you may just see the bonds among your family members strengthening. For example, because diabetes puts families on a more rigid schedule, many end up spending more time together. Susan Briston, whose son David was diagnosed as a toddler, recalled that when he was too young to understand *why* he had to eat all his food, the family would "sit and talk at the dinner table until he was able to finish." Most families haven't done that since the good old "Leave It to Beaver" days — and many wish they *did!*

The bottom line on all this? You have to make a choice: You can let diabetes pull you apart, or you can pull together as a family, against it. Like many other families, we've found that our involvement in the Juvenile Diabetes Foundation has helped us pull together. It's allowed us to turn our energies outward. It's given us a positive way to channel our hopes for Casey's future and the future of millions of kids like her, all around the world. We hope your family will join ours and all the others like us not only in *hoping* for a cure, but in *working* toward it.

A F T E R W O R D

Kenneth Farber
Executive Director,
Juvenile Diabetes Foundation International

Four years ago, the Juvenile Diabetes Foundation named the 1990s JDF's "Decade for the Cure." We were optimistic then, and we have even more reason to be excited now.

The most important news of the decade to date, without a doubt, was the publication in June of 1993, of the Diabetes Control and Complications Trial, or DCCT. The DCCT was a large scale, multi-year study of over one thousand diabetic patients, to determine the relationship between blood sugar control and diabetic complications. Physicians have long suspected that the two are related, but this was the first large scale study to document the specific relationship between blood sugars at varying levels and risk for specific complications.

The DCCT demonstrated conclusively that controlling blood sugar matters—and that it matters a lot. Those patients who meticulously regulate their blood sugar levels are at lower risk for diabetic retinopathy (which can lead to blindness—the most feared diabetic complication) and for diabetic nephropathy, or kidney disease, the most lethal risk of diabetes.

The conclusive evidence that controlling blood sugar levels can lower the risk of complications is good news not only for medical reasons, but for psychological reasons as well: Diabetes no longer has to instill in its victims a sense of hopelessness. There are things — specific things — people with diabetes can do to control their blood sugar, and doing those things can help you live a longer and much healthier life.

Happily, we may be closer to a big breakthrough that will make that blood sugar control far easier: the development of noninvasive blood glucose monitors. To keep your blood sugar as close to normal as possible without lowering it too far and running the risk of hypoglycemia, it's best to test your blood sugar many times over the course of the day. But how many times a day does anyone want to prick his or her own finger and draw blood?

Today, several research groups and manufacturers are perfecting noninvasive blood glucose monitors. When available, these devices will allow diabetics to test their blood glucose levels in seconds, using infra-red technology instead of drawing blood. You'll be able to put your finger or arm on a pad or in a sensor, in the path of a light wave, and have a digital read-out in seconds. Work on these monitors is progressing rapidly. Given the degree to which noninvasive monitors will simplify life with diabetes, it's no exaggeration to say that their perfection will be the single greatest advance in diabetes science and care since the discovery of insulin back in the 1920s.

And while the JDF is funding research that will make living with diabetes easier, we are also devoting great attention to research that will one day make it possible to live without diabetes, altogether.

Our hopes of eradicating diabetes aren't based on wishful thinking, but on logical thinking: If you look at the history of medical research in the twentieth century you will see three different classes of disease that scientists have approached. The first two have already seen dramatic progress. With antibiotics, doctors can now treat many bacterial diseases that were once life threatening. Similarly, scientists have almost eradicated a whole class of viral diseases, like measles, mumps and polio, with vaccines. Once epidemic, these diseases have also become dim memories in most industrialized countries, except for the outbreaks that occur when people become lax about vaccinations.

Today, we are hopeful that a third class of diseases, the autoimmune diseases, will soon be as vague a memory as the bacterial and viral diseases that once plagued our society. This last class of diseases includes Type-I diabetes, rheumatoid arthritis, lupus and multiple sclerosis, which are all characterized by the body's immune system attacking a part of itself. The difference among these diseases is the *part* of the body being attacked. If it is the beta cells, which produce insulin, one develops Type-I diabetes; if it is the joints, arthritis results. And while the symptoms of these diseases differ greatly, the similarity in their origins means that once scientists learn how to manipulate the immune system and stop it from attacking the human body, they may also be able to defeat all of these diseases.

As diabetologists continue to work with researchers in other fields, they are also working vigorously on the problems of diabetes itself: on preventing the disease in the first place, on curing those who have it, and on curing the complications that arise in long-term diabetics.

Preventing diabetes is very important for two reasons: We want not only to prevent anyone else from getting diabetes, but also to ensure that the people we hope to cure in the future don't develop diabetes all over again.

In order to prevent Type-I diabetes, scientists have been studying the factors that cause it. Today we know that there are three factors that conspire to make a person diabetic: First, he or she must have a genetic susceptibility to the disease. The second factor in developing Type-I diabetes is a trigger mechanism, which may be a virus. Many children develop diabetes after a bout of the chicken pox or flu. This happens too often to be sheer coincidence, and scientists are researching the connections between viruses and diabetes in an effort to break the cause-and-effect chain that links them in genetically susceptible children.

Environmental factors may also trigger diabetes. Some scientists are suggesting that chemical pollutants or stress may be triggers. Other scientists have suggested that bacterial infections can bring on diabetes in those whose genes are "programmed" for it. While none of these factors can *cause* diabetes in a child without genetic predisposition, they may allow the diabetes to manifest itself.

The third step in the development of Type-I diabetes is what we call an auto-immune destructive process. The body is no longer able to recognize its own insulin-producing tissue as part of itself, so it dispatches its immune system to the pancreas and destroys the insulin-producing islets. When enough insulin-producing tissue is destroyed, diabetes results.

Under the auspices of the Juvenile Diabetes Foundation, scientists have spent twenty years and many millions of dollars trying to understand how diabetes develops. Now that we understand why diabetes develops and how children *get* diabetes, we can begin searching for ways to eradicate it and to prevent it in the future.

To help find those answers, scientists are exploring ways of altering the genetic susceptibility to diabetes. If we could find out who is susceptible and alter that susceptibility, we could prevent diabetes. Scientists have already identified which component of a person's genetic system teaches the body's immune system to recognize self from nonself. The specific genes that cause diabetes have not been found as of this writing, but we are looking very vigorously for them. Once we have identified the gene that causes autoimmune diseases, we will be able to work on repairing the defective genes in people at risk for diabetes.

Researchers are looking for ways to protect diabetes-susceptible patients from the trigger mechanisms (by vaccinating against trigger viruses, for example). If we could do that, it is possible that the diabetes would never manifest itself.

Scientists are also trying to figure out ways to manipulate the immune system. They have spent a great deal of time figuring out what the immunological problems of diabetes are, and as a result of their efforts, we are ready to *solve* those problems.

To do that, we must first identify the target on the beta cell that inspires this attack of the immune system. Second, we must discover what part of the immune system is killing the insulin-producing cell.

We are especially optimistic about the fact that scientists are beginning to identify which parts of the immune system are attacking the beta cells. Many researchers are focusing on a specific type of immune cell called lymphocytes, which produce powerful "killing" chemicals called lymphokines. (You may have heard of lymphokines, the group that includes cancer drugs like interferon and interluken #1.) Some scientists think that these chemicals kill the pancreatic beta cells. If we can figure out whether—and if so, which—lymphokines are responsible, then perhaps we could neutralize them without harming the rest of the immune system.

Though this concept sounds like science fiction, it is well rooted in reality. We already know that Type-I diabetes is a preventable disease. A significant percentage of newly diagnosed diabetic patients using general immunosuppressive drugs like cyclosporin (a drug used to prevent transplant rejection) can prevent diabetes from progressing. Unfortunately, cyclosporin is a potent drug that leaves the patient open to risk of kidney damage, infection, and cancers. Therefore, most physicians don't think cyclosporin is an appropriate drug for diabetic children who are otherwise healthy.

But even if cyclosporin is not the answer, knowing how it works in preventing the progression of diabetes helps us identify an important goal: Our challenge today is to find drugs that have all of cyclosporin's advantages without its disadvantages.

Like those focusing on prevention, scientists focusing on curing diabetes have already gathered much of the raw data they will need in order to progress. In the past decade or so, they have confirmed that Type-I diabetes is conceptually a very simple disease: the beta cells are destroyed by the immune system, and they don't produce insulin, which the body needs to turn food into energy. As a result of that understanding, we know that to cure diabetes or at least treat it more effectively, we must deliver insulin into non-insulin-producing bodies.

Since Drs. Banting and Best discovered insulin in 1921, diabetics have injected it into their bodies a few times every day. Unfortunately, one, two or three shots a day do not mimic the exquisite process that occurs in a healthy pancreas. Therefore, we must determine better ways to deliver insulin to non-insulin-producing bodies.

There are several possibilities: One is increasing the number of injections. Giving four, five or six injections of insulin a day would be somewhat more akin to how a normal pancreas produces the hormone, but it still would not be identical. Another option is the insulin pump — a mechanical device that sends insulin into the body at a preprogrammed rate, with adjustments at mealtimes and at night. This is better than individual shots, but it still does not adequately replace a healthy pancreas, because the device cannot read the blood sugar level the way a pancreas would and regulate the amount of insulin precisely. Researchers are currently trying to improve the insulin pump by attaching the kind of noninvasive sensor described earlier in this chapter, to govern the release of insulin based precisely on the body's minute-by-minute needs.

Toward the ultimate goal of making insulin shots or pumps completely obsolete, doctors are attempting islet-cell-transplants; if bodies that do not produce their own insulin could receive — and retain — transplanted cells to do the job for them, diabetes would be cured . . . or at least, tremendously alleviated. But as simple as it sounds, transplanting pancreases is very complex. For one thing, a transplant requires major surgery and immunosuppressive drugs that have serious side effects. Secondly, given the difficulty of finding enough hearts, lungs and livers for *those* organ transplants, we have no reason to believe that there would ever be enough organs available to help the millions of diabetics who would need them.

Therefore, scientists are studying alternative ways to cure diabetes by transplanting just the islet cells, instead of entire pancreases. Surgeons have, indeed, successfully transplanted islet cells into some diabetic patients, and while most of those patients are still immunosuppressed, some are off insulin — which in itself is quite remarkable.

To eliminate the need for immunosuppression, scientists are looking at ways to transplant islet cells while leaving them invulnerable to recipient rejection. The most promising possibility on that front is microencapsulation: wrapping the islet cells in a membrane that would allow the insulin out into the body to do its job, without letting rejection cells in to destroy the transplanted cells.

So far, this has only been done in a few patients, but it may be working, which gives us great hope: If microencapsulating islet cells keeps them protected and functioning, we might be able to use animal tissue. As we know from 50 years of success with porcine insulin before human insulin was available for injection, pig insulin and human insulins are very similar. If we can microencapsulate and transplant pig islets, we will solve the transplant rejection problem and the islet source problem concurrently.

Another approach to curing diabetes is the possibility of creating a surrogate beta cell. There is some preliminary evidence that we may be able to get other cells in the body to produce insulin using genetic engineering techniques. Of course, learning how to manipulate the cells in that way is only half the challenge; the goal is not to produce insulin incessantly, but to create a system within which insulin is regulated by blood sugar, as it is in healthy bodies.

These are just some of the studies JDF is funding in our fight against diabetes. We are confident that in the next decade or so, one or more of them will be developed to the point that it can help us eradicate the disease, or at least make it less destructive. In the meantime, JDF also has a commitment to enhancing and easing the lives of current diabetics and reducing the disease's complications, as well as the fear those complications often cause.

While it would be inaccurate to say that the *only* thing diabetics have to fear is fear itself, the fear of complications *can* often affect a diabetic's life as adversely as the complications themselves. From the moment their doctors tell them about the risk of blindness, kidney failure, and amputations, many diabetics live in dread that they will develop these complications. In some ways, the dread can be worse than the complications themselves. For unlike the complications that may never set in at all or that may set in only in old age, the fear can cripple childhood and the teenage years, hanging like a dark cloud over the diabetic's life. Therefore, our research into curing diabetes' complications is an attempt not only to help diabetics live *longer* lives, but to help them live happier less stressful lives as well.

The risk of complications has already diminished significantly by advances in blood sugar control. As scientists gain greater understanding of the relationship between blood-sugar levels and diabetic complications, they will be able to limit dramatically the incidence of these complications.

One hypothesis is that the sugar in a diabetic's blood attaches to protein and forms a substance like Krazy Glue, which adheres to the inside of blood vessels. The substance traps all kind of material (like cholesterol) that is circulating in the bloodstream, which can ultimately damage the artery, and impair circulation to target organs like the eyes or kidneys. Understanding how this bodily adhesive works may ultimately lead us to a therapy. If we could develop drugs that inhibit the coupling of glucose and protein to form the substance, the blood vessels would not clog, and ultimately the target organs would not be damaged.

In addition to developing new drugs, scientists are exploring ways in which medications already available to treat other diseases can help slow the course of diabetic complications. In the summer of 1993, The Bristol-Myers Squibb company announced findings that Capoten, a drug used routinely to control blood pressure, can also reduce kidney disease in diabetics. Patients who had early warning signs of diabetic nephropathy and took Capoten significantly lowered their risk of developing severe diabetic nephropathy.

Reading through this chapter, you have probably noticed a theme: Scientists can only figure out a therapy when they understand the root of the problem. Until we knew exactly what causes diabetes, we could not prevent it. But now that we do understand what causes the disease, we have opened up a world of options, bringing hope to millions of diabetics.

Since a small cadre of parents founded the Juvenile Diabetes Foundation 24 years ago, we have spent over $150 million to develop a tremendous amount of preliminary data. We are now poised to put that data together in a very meaningful way. Biomedical research is much like building a house: You start with the foundation, and then the walls go up. Finally, the roof goes on, and only then are you ready to move in — to zero in on the ways to prevent diabetes, to cure it, and to treat it . . . to hone in on the right questions, so we can ask them and get the right answers.

We are already turning data into life-altering results. We are on the verge of having of having a very dramatic impact on the complications of diabetes, and I think we are entering an age when the complications of diabetes will be largely controllable. Actually curing the disease will be somewhat more difficult, but I am confident that will happen, too, before very long, especially if research is adequately funded.

Along these lines, JDF has launched an International Initiative, "The Only Remedy Is A Cure," with the goal of raising $100 million for diabetes research. The cornerstone of this initiative is its "Programs of Excellence" grants program, which teams world class scientists who specialize in diabetes research with scientists in such burgeoning areas of biomedical research as immunology, molecular biology, and genetics. It is an extraordinary effort to move diabetes research many steps closer to a cure. Wide-ranging programs like this are ambitious and very costly . . . and that's one reason we need *you*. The Juvenile Diabetes Foundation needs every person and family whose life is touched by diabetes to join us not only in hoping for a cure, but in working toward it. Your local JDF chapter needs your support to raise the funds that will cure the disease. And we are there to offer *you* support as well, through our programs and literature and membership activities.

Through the Juvenile Diabetes Foundation, you can learn about advances in diabetes treatment and about the progress we are making toward a cure. In addition to the support and information we can offer you, we have something else to share: our optimism.

There is a cure for diabetes. And together, we will find it.

APPENDIX A

Further Reading and Information

BOOKS

Parenting a Diabetic Child. By Gloria Loring. This book offers excellent insights as well as reassurance for parents of the newly diagnosed child. In simple terms, it focuses on explaining the disease, caring for your child, and evaluating diabetes professionals. The book concludes with a research update and a resource section that are very helpful and informative.

Diabetes: A New and Complete Guide to Healthier Living for Parents, Children and Young Adults Who Have Insulin-Dependent Diabetes. By Lee Ducat and Sherry Suib Cohen. This is indeed a practical guide to living with diabetes, written by the founder of the Juvenile Diabetes Foundation. Its information, recommendations, and first-hand experiences were very helpful to us in learning to cope with the problems and demands of diabetes.

Take This Book To the Hospital With You: A Consumer Guide To Surviving Your Hospital Stay. By Charles B. Inlander and Ed Weiner. Pantheon Books. Provides the information and encouragement you need to get the best possible care in the hospital.

An Instructional Aid on Insulin-Dependent Diabetes Mellitus. By Luther B. Travis, M.D., F.A.A.P. Children's Diabetes Management Center, Dept. of Pediatrics. The University of Texas Medical Branch, Galveston, Texas. We found this workbook incredibly helpful right after Casey was diagnosed. In addition to clarifying diabetes-management information, the book provides quizzes so that you and your child can make sure you *understand* the information well enough to put it into practice.

139

Families: Crisis and Caring. By T. Berry Brazelton, M.D. Ballantine. Includes chapters on dealing with a chronic illness, as well
as general information on coping with circumstances that place
a strain on your family.

*Meeting the Challenge of Disability or Chronic Illness — A Family
Guide.* By Lori A. Goldfarb, Mary Jane Brothers, Jean Ann Summers, and Ann P. Turnbull. Brookes. Includes step-by-step
methods to identify, prevent, and solve problems caused by
child's chronic illness.

If Your Child Has Diabetes. By Joanne Elliott. Perigee. Arranged in
easy-to-read question/answer format, this book is a handy reference for specific diabetes-related facts and issues.

ORGANIZATIONS

Juvenile Diabetes Foundation International
The Diabetes Research Foundation
432 Park Avenue South
New York, NY 10016
800-JDF-CURE
212-889-7575
The Juvenile Diabetes Foundation International gives more money
directly to diabetes research than any other non-governmental
health agency in the world. Among its public information services,
it provides brochures and a toll-free diabetes information line:
800-JDF-CURE.
To order JDF's quarterly research publication, *Countdown,* and
become a member of JDF, write to JDF at 432 Park Ave. S., New
York, NY 10016.

American Diabetes Association
1660 Duke Street
Alexandria, VA 22314
800-ADA-DISC

Offers support groups, newsletters, and a magazine, *Diabetes Forecast.*

To order ADA's Buyers Guide to Diabetes Products, send $3.75 check to ADA

1970 Chain Bridge Rd.

McLean, VA 22109

National Diabetes Information Clearinghouse

Box NDIC

Bethesda, MD 20205

301-468-2162

Will provide you with pamphlets and newsletters, and will help you search for general and specific information about diabetes.

Association for the Care of Children's Health

3615 Wisconsin Avenue N.W.

Washington, DC 20202

Will send you info on health insurance; write to them at the address above to request a pamphlet.

National Center for Youth with Disabilities

University of Minnesota

Box 721-UMHC

Harvard Street at East River Road

Minneapolis, MN 55455

800-333-6293

Will do customized computer searches and compile bibliographies of diabetes-related journal articles for you for a small fee. The Center also publishes newsletters and sponsors conferences about topics related to chronic illnesses in children and teens.

Sibling Information Network

The A.J. Pappanikou Center on Special Education and Rehabilitation

991 Main Street

East Hartford, CT 06108

203-282-7050

Though primarily geared to siblings of physically and mentally handicapped children, this group does produce some literature and videotapes of interest to the brothers and sisters of diabetics.

The Diabetes Research Center at Indiana University Medical Center
Will provide you with free guidelines on exercise and sports-training for diabetics. Call 317-630-6370.

Children's Diabetes Center in Milwaukee
Offers intensive courses and seminars for newly diagnosed diabetics and their families. For more information, call 608-262-9300.

The American Association of Diabetes Educators
500 N. Michigan Ave.
Suite 1400
Chicago, IL 60601
312-661-1700
Can provide a list of Certified Diabetes Educators in your area.

American Dietetic Association
216 W. Jackson Blvd.
Suite 800
Chicago, IL 60606
312-899-0040
Will provide the names and phone numbers of registered dieticians in your area.

Barbara Davis Center for Childhood Diabetes
To contact the Barbara Davis Center, mentioned in Chapter 3, call 303-623-2873. The Center provides care and conducts research, and has treated patients from around the world.

Diabetes Treatment Centers of America
1 Burton Hills Blvd.
Nashville, TN 37215
800-327-DTCA
Will give you list of centers in your area, or will help you identify the center closest to where you live.

SugarFree Centers for Diabetics
13715 Burbank Blvd.
P.O. Box 114
Van Nuys, CA 91408
800-972-2323, or in California, 800-336-1222
A resource for cookbooks, pamphlets, and sugar-free foods.

Joslin Diabetes Center
One Joslin Place
Boston, MA 02215
617-732-2400
(See expanded listings in Appendix C, starting on page 147.)

APPENDIX B

Diabetes Supply Houses

Listed below are vendors who offer supplies at fairly low prices —
many below retail. To get the best value, request a catalog or listing
of their supplies, and you will be able to comparison shop.

Bruce Medical Supply
441 Waverly Oaks Road
Waltham, MA 02254
Phone 800-225-8446
Call in Massachusetts
800-342-8955.

Diabetes Center Pharmacy
P.O. Box 739
Wayzata, MN 55391
Phone 800-848-2793
Collect in Minnesota
612-541-0239

Diabetes Cost Club
450 S. Gravers Road
Plymouth Meeting, PA
    19462
Phone 800-288-9980
or 215-275-1325

Diabetic Express
P.O. Box 80037
Canton, OH 44708
Phone 800-338-4656

Diabetes Supply Centers of
    America
P.O. Box 101486
Nashville, TN 37210
Phone 800-422-0444
Collect in Tennessee
615-889-6123

Home Service Medical
P.O. Box 4603
Minneapolis, MN 55446
Phone 800-888-5651

H-8 Medical Supplies
P.O. Box 42
Whitehall, PA 18052
Phone 800-344-7633

Thriftee Pharmacy & Home
    Diabetes Care
P.O. Box 12568
Roanoke, VA 24026
Phone 800-847-4383
or 703-989-1249

APPENDIX C

Diabetes Treatment and Education Centers

ADA-ACCREDITED CENTERS

Following is a list of diabetes education and treatment centers accredited by the American Diabetes Association. Those marked with an asterisk* have special programs for treating and educating children.

Alabama

Lloyd Noland Hospital
Diabetes Education
  Program
701 Lloyd Noland Parkway
Fairfield, AL 35064
Brian Beckett, PharmD

Providence Hospital
The Diabetes Center
6801 Airport Boulevard
Mobile, AL 36685
Edward Walters, EdD

University of Alabama at
  Birmingham
Diabetes Research & Educ.
  Hospital
Room D-112
1808 7th Ave. South

Birmingham, AL 35233
Valerie Crenshaw, RN

Arizona

CIGNA Healthplan of
  Arizona
Outpatient Diabetes
  Program
755 East McDowell Road
Phoenix, AZ 85006
Phyllis Salem, MS, RD,
  CDE

Carondolet St. Joseph's
  Hospital
Diabetes Care Center
350 N. Wilmot Road
Tucson, AZ 85711
Patricia M. Hiller, RN,
  MEd, CDE

California

Cedars-Sinai Medical
Center
Diabetes Outpatient
Training and Education
Center (DOTEC)
8730 Beverly Blvd.
Room 134 E. Plaza
Los Angeles, CA 90048
Mary A. Pearce, RN, MS,
CDE

Daniel Freeman Hospitals,
Inc.
Diabetes Care Center
333 North Prairie
Inglewood, CA 90301
Julie Oldenburg, RD, CDE

Eisenhower Memorial
Hospital
The Diabetes Program
Probst Suite 100
39000 Bob Hope Drive
Rancho Mirage, CA 92270
Patricia Granuci, RN

John Muir Medical Center
Diabetes Center
112 La Casa Via, Suite 210
Walnut Creek, CA 94598
Judy Kohn, RN

Little Company of Mary
Hospital
Diabetes Management
Program
4101 Torrance Blvd.

Torrance, CA 90503
Nancy Tsuyuki, RN

Loma Linda University
Medical Center
Diabetes Treatment Center
11255 Mt. View Avenue
Suite I
Loma Linda, CA 92354
Ila M. Spangler

Mercy Hospital and
Medical Center
Diabetes Education Program
4077 Fifth Avenue
San Diego, CA 92103-2180
Sandra Winter, RN, MSN,
CDE

Mercy San Juan Hospital
Diabetes Center
6501 Coyle Avenue
Carmichael, CA 95608
Carol Anders, RN, MS

Mt. Diablo Medical Center
Center for Diabetes
2222 East Street, Suite 280
Concord, CA 94520
Marloe Campbell, RN

Parkview Community
Hospital
Diabetes Treatment Centers
of America
3865 Jackson Street
Riverside, CA 92503
Charlotte Hodge, RN, NP,
CDE

St. Jude Hospital &
  Rehabilitation Center
The Diabetes Life Center
101 E. Valencia Mesa Drive
Fullerton, CA 92635
Beatrice Schultz, RN

Scripps Memorial·
  Hospital–Chula Vista
534 H Street
Chula Vista, CA 92012
Louise Rahmann, RN,
  CDE

Sharp Cabrillo Hospital
Diabetes Center
3475 Kenyon Street
San Diego, CA 92110
Jacqui Thompson, RN

Sutter General Hospital
Sutter Diabetes Care Center
2801 L Street
Sacramento, CA 95816
Susan Gaston, RN, MN

Tarzana Regional Medical
  Center
Diabetes Treatment Centers
  of America
18321 Clark Street
Tarzana, CA 91356
Donna Bender, BA

Warrack Hospital
2449 Summerfield Road
Santa Rosa, CA 95405
Macbeth Moser, RN,
  CDE

Colorado

Rose Medical Center
Diabetes Treatment Centers
  of America
4567 East Ninth Avenue
Denver, CO 80220
Karen Lollar, RN, MBA,
  CDE

Connecticut

Hartford Hospital
Diabetes Life Care
80 Seymour Street
Hartford, CT 06115
Anita Gorman, RN

St. Francis Hospital and
  Medical Center
Diabetes Care Center
114 Woodland Street
Hartford, CT 06105
Nicholas Abourizk, MD

District of Columbia

Greater Southeast
  Community Hospital
Diabetes in Control
  Management Program
1310 Southern Avenue S.E.
Washington, DC 20032
William Driskill, RN, CDE

Walter Reed Army Medical
  Center
Diabetes Education
  Program

Washington, DC
20307-5001
Stephen Clement, MD,
CDE

Florida

Baptist Hospital Diabetes
Education Center
910 West Blount Street
Pensacola, FL 32501
Anita King, RN, MA, CDE

Baptist Hospital of Miami
The Diabetes Care Program
8900 North Kendall Drive
Miami, FL 33176-2197
Lois Exelbert, RN, MS,
CDE

Coral Gables Hospital
Diabetes Education
Program
3100 Douglas Road
Coral Gables, FL 33134
Jane L. Sparrow, RN, CDE

Florida Hospital Medical
Center
601 East Rollins Street
Orlando, FL 32803
Beth Kraas, ARNP, MSN,
CDE

Joslin Diabetes Clinic
Memorial Medical Center
of Jacksonville
3627 University Blvd.
South

Suite 435
Jacksonville, FL 32216
Kathy Zoumberis, RN, CDE

Lee Memorial Hospital
Diabetes Treatment Centers
of America
2776 Cleveland Avenue
Fort Myers, FL 33901
Valerie Barr, RN, BS

Mease Health Care
833 Milwaukee Avenue
P.O. Box 760
Dunedin, FL 34296-0760
Polly Meadows, RN,
CDE

Methodist Medical Center
Diabetes Treatment Centers
of America
580 W. Eighth Street
Jacksonville, FL 32209
Virginia Schenzinger, RN,
MN, CDE

North Ridge Medical
Center
Diabetes Treatment Centers
of America
5757 N. Dixie Hwy.
Ft. Lauderdale, FL 33334
Sarah Schroeder

Orlando Regional Medical
Center
Diabetes Treatment Centers
of America
1414 South Kuhe Avenue

Orlando, FL 32806-2093
Cynthia Healy, RN, BSN,
    CDE

University Community
    Hospital
Diabetes Treatment Centers
    of America
3100 East Fletcher Avenue
Tampa, FL 33613
Al Tudene, CDE

University of Miami
    Diabetes Diagnostic and
    Treatment Center
1500 NW 12th Avenue
Suite 900
Miami, FL 33136
Della Matheson, RN, CDE

West Florida Medical Center
Diabetes Management
    Center
8383 N. Davis Hwy.
Pensacola, FL 32514
Joy Darby, MS, RD

Georgia

Candler General Hospital
Diabetes Education
    Program
5353 Reynolds Street
Savannah, GA 31405
Lisa Goodwin, RN, CDE

The Emory Clinic
Section of Internal
    Medicine

1365 Clifton Road, N.E.
Atlanta, GA 30322
Gayle Russo, RN, MN, CDE

Georgia Center for Diabetes
4470 N. Shallowford Road
Suite 101
Atlanta, GA 30338
Thomas Flood, MD

Humana Hospital-Augusta
Diabetes Care Center
3651 Wheeler Road
Augusta, GA 30910
Carol Pardue, RN, MSN,
    CDE

Hutcheson Medical Center
100 Gross Crescent Circle
Fort Oglethorpe, GA 30742
Betsy Piloian, RN, MSN,
    CDE

South Georgia Medical
    Center
P.O. Box 1727
Valdosta, GA 31601-1727
Linda Wiseman, RN, CDE

University Hospital
1350 Walton Way
Augusta, GA 30910-3599
Sara Brodie, RN, CDE

Hawaii

Straub Clinic and Hospital
The Diabetes Center of the
    Pacific
888 South King Street

Honolulu, HI 96813
Alice Taniguchi, RN, MPH,
    CDE

Illinois

Carle Clinic Association
602 West University
    Avenue
Urbana, IL 61801
Sandra Burke, MSN, RNC,
    CDE

Glen Ellyn Clinic, SC
Diabetes Education
    Program
454 Pennsylvania Avenue
Glen Ellyn, IL 60137
Jacqueline Tack, RN,
    CDE

Highland Park Hospital
718 Glenview Avenue
Highland Park, IL 60035
Margaret Carpentier, BSN

Holy Family Hospital
Stable Lives Diabetes
    Program
100 N. River Road
Des Plaines, IL 60016
Donald Uhlmeyer

St. Francis of Evanston
Diabetes Treatment Centers
    of America
355 Ridge Avenue
Evanston, IL 60202
Margaret A. Greco

Office of Gerald Sobel, MD
111 North Wabash Avenue
Chicago, IL 60602
Monica Joyce, RD, CDE

Springfield Diabetes &
    Endocrine Center
"Take Charge of Your
    Diabetes"
2528 Farragut Drive
Springfield, IL 62704
Anne Daly, RD, MS, CDE

VA Medical Center–North
    Chicago
Endocrine/Metabolic
    Section (111E)
3001 Greenbay Road
North Chicago, IL 60064
Janine Stoll, RN, CDE

Indiana

Lafayette Home Hospital
Regional Diabetes Center
2400 South Street
Lafayette IN 47904
Sally A. Stacey, RN

Parkview Regional
Diabetes Care Center
2200 Randallia Drive
Fort Wayne, IN 46805
Nancy Andrews, RN, CDE

St. Joseph Hospital
Taking Charge of Your
    Diabetes
215 West Fourth Street

Mishawaka, IN 46544
Sister Sharon Marie Fox,
   RN, BSN, CDE

St. Margaret Hospital and
   Health Centers
Adult Diabetes Education
   Program
5454 Hohman Avenue
Hammond, IN 46320
Dorothy Klapak, RN, MS

Iowa

Allen Memorial Hospital
International Diabetes
   Center–North
Iowa Affiliate
1825 Logan Avenue
Waterloo, IA 50703
Sandra Thrum, RN, BSN,
   CDE

Covenant Medical Center
3421 W. Ninth Street and
   2101 Kimball Avenue
Waterloo, IA 50702
Rachel Jenson, RN

McFarland Diabetes Center
1215 Duff Avenue
Ames, IA 50010
Charlene Freeman, RN, CDE

*University of Iowa
   Hospitals and Clinics
   (UIHC)
Diabetes-Endocrinology
   Unit

Iowa City, IA 52242
Vicki L. Kraus, MS, RN,
   CDE

Kansas

Bethany Medical Center
Diabetes Education Program
51 North 12th Street
Kansas City, KS 66102
Jamie Lawson, RN, CDE

Stormont-Vail Regional
   Medical Center
Diabetes Learning Center
1500 W. 10th Street
Topeka, KS 66604
Christine Clarkin, RNC,
   CDE

*St. Joseph Medical Center
3600 E. Harry
Wichita, KS 67218
Deborah Hinnen, RN, MN,
   CDE

Kentucky

Humana
   Hospital–Lexington
150 North Eagle Creek
   Drive
Lexington, KY 40509
Cindy Thompson

Lourdes Hospital
Diabetes Patient Education
   Program
1530 Lone Oak Road

Paducah, KY 42003
Sophia Chandler, RN, CDE

Mercy Hospital
Diabetes Education
  Program
1006 Ford Avenue
Owensboro, KY 42301
Rosemary Craig, RN

Methodist Evangelical
  Hospital
Diabetes Care Center
315 E. Broadway
Louisville, KY 40202-1703
Sara Crawford, RN, CDE

Northern Kentucky
  Diabetes
  Control Program
401 Park Avenue
Newport, KY 41071
Patricia Foxworthy, RD,
  MS

St. Luke Hospital East
Diabetes Center
85 North Grand Avenue
Fort Thomas, KY 41075
Benita Burgess, BSN
(606) 572-3400

Saints Mary & Elizabeth
  Hospital
Diabetes Treatment Centers
  of America
1850 Bluegrass Avenue
Louisville, KY 40215
Paula Pierce, RD, CDE

Louisiana

Baton Rouge General
  Medical Center
The Diabetes Center
3600 Florida Boulevard
Baton Rouge, LA
  70821-2511
Peggy Bourgeois, RN, BSN,
  CDE

East Jefferson General
  Hospital
Diabetes Management
  Center
4200 Houma Blvd.
Metairie, LA 70011
Anne Buescher, RN, CDE

Glenwood Regional
  Medical Center
Diabetes Treatment Centers
  of America
P.O. Box 35805
West Monroe, LA
  71294-5805
Frances McGough

Medical Center of Baton
  Rouge
Diabetes Management
  Center
17000 Medical Center Drive
Baton Rouge, LA 70816
Pam Bassett, MS, RD, LDN

Diabetes Center of
  North Monroe Hospital
3421 Medical Park Drive

Monroe, LA 71203
Richard Huth

St. Francis Medical Center
Diabetes Care Center
309 Jackson Street
Monroe, LA 71201
Janis Webber, RN

Tulane University Medical
    Center
Center for Diabetes
1415 Tulane Avenue
New Orleans, LA 70112
Trudy Parker, RN,
    CDE

Willis-Knighton Medical
    Center
2600 Greenwood Road
Shreveport, LA 71103
Frances Hazzard, LDN,
    RD

Maine

Cary Medical Center
37 Van Buren Road
Caribou, ME 04736
Gloria Bouchard, RN

Eastern Maine Medical
    Center
"Managing Your Diabetes"
489 State Street
Bangor, ME 04401
Pat Stenger, RN, CDE

Yankee Healthcare, Inc.
152 Dresden Avenue

P.O. Box 550
Gardner, ME 04345
Kathleen Beers, RN

Maryland

Suburban Hospital
8600 Old Georgetown
    Road
Bethesda, MD 20814
Joan Wells, RN, CDE

Massachusetts

Baystate Medical Center
Diabetes Teaching
    Program
759 Chestnut Street
Springfield, MA 01199
Darlene Biggs, RN, MSN,
    CDE

*Joslin Diabetes
    Center
One Joslin Place
Boston, MA 02215
Donna Richardson, RN,
    MS, CDE
(See expanded list, page
    171.)

Waltham Weston Hospital
    & Medical Center
Diabetes Treatment Centers
    of America
5 Hope Avenue
Waltham, MA 02254-9116
Debra Kaplan

Michigan

Henry Ford Hospital
Ambulatory Diabetes
Regulation/Education
  Program
2799 West Grand Blvd.
Detroit, MI 48202
Iris J. Whitehouse, RN,
  BSN, CDE

MidMichigan Regional
  Medical Center
International Diabetes
  Center Affiliate
4005 Orchard Drive
Midland, MI 48670
Marilyn Haeussler

Minnesota

Duluth Diabetes Center
404 East 4th Street
Duluth, MN 55805
Gwen Hall-Verchota, RN,
  MA, CDE

Fairview Southdale
  Hospital
Diabetes Education and
  Self- Management
  Program
6401 France Avenue South
Edina, MN 55435
Karen Mecklenberg, RN,
  MSN

Group Health, Inc.
Diabetes Education Program

22829 University Avenue
  S.E.
Minneapolis, MN 55414
Carolé Mensing, RN, MA

*International Diabetes
  Center
Park Nicollet Medical
  Foundation
5000 West 39th Street
Minneapolis, MN 55416
Judy Ostrom Joynes, RN,
  MA, CDE

Mayo Clinic
Diabetes Clinic, N15
200 First Street S.W.
Rochester, MN 55905
Naomi Munene, RN

North Memorial Medical
  Center
Diabetes Education
  Program
3300 North Oakdale
Robbinsdale, MN 55422
Melissa Kiefer, RN

Rice Memorial Hospital
IDC-Willmar Associate
301 Becker Avenue
  S.W.
Willmar, MN 56201
Deborah Lippert

St. Luke's Hospital
Diabetes Education
  Program
915 East First Street

Duluth, MN 55805
Cristine Stephenson

Missouri

*Barnes Hospital
Diabetes Education
   Program
One Barnes Hospital Plaza
St. Louis, MO 63110
Patricia Potter, RN, MSN

*Children's Mercy Hospital
824th at Gillham Road
Kansas City, MO 64108
Joyce Mosiman, RD, CDE

Cox Diabetes Center
Lester E. Cox Medical
   Centers
1423 N. Jefferson
Springfield, MO 65802
Shirley Phillips, RN

International Diabetes
   Center
Kansas City Regional
   Affiliate
2184 East Meyer Blvd.
Kansas City, MO 64132
Mary Fulton, RN, BA, CDE

Lucy Lee Hospital
Diabetes Education
   Program
2620 N. Westwood Blvd.
Poplar Bluff, MO 63901
Jolene Kotschwar, RN,
   MSN

St. John's Mercy Medical
   Center
615 South Ballas Road
St. Louis, MO 63141-8221
Katie Stewart, RN, CDE

St. John's Regional Health
   Center
Diabetes Education Series
1235 E. Cherokee
Springfield, MO 65804-2263
Yvonne Morris, RN, CDE

St. Luke's Hospital
Diabetes Center
Peet Outpatient Center
Warnall Road at 44th
Kansas City, MO 64111
Ruth Mencl, RN, MN, CDE

St. Mary's Health Center
Diabetes Education Program
6420 Clayton Road
St. Louis, MO 63117
Marie Campbell, RN, BSN

Trinity Lutheran Hospital
Diabetes Treatment Centers
   of America
3030 Baltimore
Kansas City, MO 64108
Mary Frances Haake, BA

Montana

Trinity Hospital
Outpatient Education
   Program
315 Knapp Street

Wolf Point, MT 59102
Sandy Rensvold

Nebraska

Midlands Diabetes
  Education and Self-Help
  Center
824 Doctors Bldg., South
  Tower
4239 Farnum Road
Omaha, NE 68131
Mary Leighton, RN, BSN,
  CDE

Nevada

Desert Springs Hospital
Diabetes Education
  Program
2075 E. Flamingo Road
Las Vegas, NV 89119
Joyce Malaskovitz, RN,
  BSN, CDE

New Hampshire

St. Joseph Hospital
172 Kinsley Street
Nashua, NH 03061
Donna M. Clark, RN, BS,
  CDE

New Jersey

Diabetes Center of New
  Jersey, Inc.
1257 Marion Avenue
Plainfield, NJ 07060

Lori Sherman-Appel, RN,
  BSN, CDE

East Orange VA Medical
  Center
Diabetes Education &
  Treatment Center
Tremont Avenue
East Orange, NJ 07019
Mavourneen Mangan, MS,
  RNC, ANP, CDE

*Englewood Hospital
  Association
Diabetes Program
350 Engle Street
Englewood, NJ 07631
Nancy J. Zoebelein, RN

Monmouth Medical Center
Diabetes Treatment Center
  of America
300 Second Avenue
Long Branch, NJ 07740
Cecilia Smith-Snyder, RD,
  BS, CDE

New Mexico

Indian Health Service
Albuquerque Service Unit
801 Vassar Drive N.E.
Albuquerque, NM 87106
Lorraine Valdez, RN

New York

Diabetes Education
  Associates
600 Northern Boulevard

Suite 111
Great Neck, NY 11021
Pat McTigue, RN,
  CDE

*Mount Sinai Medical
  Center
Div. of Pediatric
  Endocrinology and
  Metabolism
One Gustave L. Levy Place
Box 1198
New York, NY 10029
Paula Liguori, RN,
  CDE

North Shore University
  Hospital
Cornell University Medical
  College
Diabetes Education &
  Treatment Center
300 Community Drive
Manhasset, NY 11030
Rita Saltiel, RN, MPH,
  CDE, CHES

St. Luke's/Roosevelt
  Hospital Center
Ambulatory Care
  Department
Amsterdam Avenue at
  114th Street
New York, NY 10025
Marjorie Clark, RN

*Winthrop-University
  Hospital
259 First Street

Mineola, NY 11501
Virginia Peragallo-Dittko,
  RN, CDE

North Carolina

The Charlotte-Mecklenburg
  Hospital Authority
Carolinas Diabetes Center
1000 Blythe Boulevard
Charlotte, NC 28207
Sue Hartman, RN, MN,
  CDE

East Carolina University
  School of Medicine
Diabetes Self-Care Program
Section of Endocrinology &
  Metabolism
Greenville, NC 27858
Sue B. Daughtry, RD, CDE

Greensboro Diabetes
  Self-Care Center
1022 Professional Village
Greensboro, NC 27401
Charles Gegick, MD

Nalle Clinic
Diabetes Center
1350 S. Kings Drive
Charlotte, NC 28207
Linda Million, RN, CDE

Raleigh Community
  Hospital
Diabetes Treatment Centers
  of America
3400 Wake Forest Road

Raleigh, NC 27609
Michael N. Tudeen

Wesley Long Community
    Hospital
Diabetes Treatment Centers
    of America
501 North Elam Avenue
P.O. Drawer X-3
Greensboro, NC 27402
Elaine Button, RN, BS,
    CDE

North Dakota

Diabetes Center MeritCare
Fargo Clinic MeritCare
737 Broadway
Fargo, ND 58123
Cheryl Stepka, MA, RN,
    CDE

Grand Forks Regional
    Diabetes Education
    Center
1000 South Columbia Road
P.O. Box 6003
Grand Forks, ND
    58206-6003
Nancy O'Connor

Ohio

Akron City Hospital
Diabetes Self-Care Program
525 East Market Street
Akron, OH 44309-2090
Kathy Jett, RN, MSN,
    CDE

*Children's Hospital
    Medical Center
Elland and Bethesda
    Avenues
Cincinnati, OH 45229-2899
Debra Drozda, RN, MS

Flower Memorial Hospital
5200 Harroun Road
Sylvania, OH 43560
Timothy J. Green

Lakewood Hospital
Diabetes Center
14519 Detroit Avenue
Lakewood, OH 44107
Joyce Bredenbeck, BSN,
    RN

Loraine Community
    Hospital
Diabetes Comprehensive
    Care Program
3700 Kolbe Road
Lorain, OH 44053-1697
Betty Mackintosh, RN, CDE

Mercy Hospital
2238 Jefferson Avenue
Toledo, OH 43624
Patti J. Gallagher, RN, CDE

Mt. Sinai Medical Center
Saltzman Institute Diabetes
    Center
University Circle
1 Mt. Sinai Drive
Cleveland, OH 44106
Eva Bradley, RN

Physicians, Inc.
Diabetes Management
    Center
825 West Market Street
Lima, OH 45011
Mary Ellen Good, MS, RN,
    CDE

Saint Thomas Medical
    Center
The Diabetes Center
444 North Main Street
Akron, OH 44310
MaryEllen Barry, RN, CDE

University MEDNET
Center for Diabetes Care
218599 Lake Shore Blvd.
Euclid, OH 44119
Karen Lenardic, RN

Oklahoma

Claremore Diabetes
    Program
U.S. Public Health Service
    Indian Hospital
101 South Moore
Claremore, OK 74017
Johnnie Brasuell, MS, RN,
    CDE

Saint Francis Hospital
Diabetes Center
William Medical Building
6585 South Yale, Suite 300
Tulsa, OK 74136
Cathey Pielsticker, RN, MS,
    CDE

Oregon

Good Samaritan Hospital &
    Medical Center
Diabetes Institute
1130 N.W. 22nd Avenue
Suite 400A
Portland, OR 97210
Joan Kono, RN

Providence Medical Center
Diabetes Treatment Centers
    of America
4805 N.E. Glisan Street
Portland, OR 97213
Patricia Oriet, RN, CDE

Salem Hospital
P.O. Box 14001
665 Winter Street S.E.
Salem, OR 97309-5014
Veralyn Klosterman, RN,
    CDE

Pennsylvania

The Chester County
    Hospital
Diabetes Learning Center
701 East Marshall Street
West Chester, PA 19380
Deborah Fitzpatrick, RN,
    CDE

*Children's Hospital of
    Pittsburgh
One Children's Place
3705 Fifth Avenue
Pittsburgh, PA 15213-2583

Jean Betschart, RN, MS,
  CDE
Linda Siminerio, RN, MS,
  CDE

*Geisinger Wyoming
  Valley Medical Center
1000 E. Mountain Drive
Wilkes-Barre, PA 18711
Roberta Hughes, RN, BS,
  CDE

Guthrie Healthcare System
Guthrie Medical Center
Guthrie Square
Sayre, PA 18840
Elizabeth Dolan, RN

Office of David Lawrence,
  MD
Education Program
  Coordinator
Internal Medicine/
  Endocrinology
301 South Seventh Avenue
West Reading, PA 19611

Montgomery Hospital
Diabetes Treatment Centers
  of America
Powell and Fornance Streets
Norristown, PA 19401
Barbara F. Pitkow, MS,
  MEd

Wilkes-Barre General
  Hospital
Diabetes Education
  Program

North River and Auburn
  Streets
Wilkes-Barre, PA 18764
Pat Ruda, RN, MNS, CDE

South Carolina

Richland Memorial
  Hospital
Diabetes Education
  Program
Five Richland Medical
  Park
Columbia, SC 29203
Kay Garrett, RN, CDE

Spartanburg Regional
  Medical Center
Diabetes Management
  Center
101 East Wood Street
Spartanburg, SC 29303
Edie McNinch

South Dakota

McKennan Hospital
Diabetes Education
  Program
800 East 21st Street
Box 5045
Sioux Falls, SD
  57117-5045
Mary Lobb, RN,
  CDE

Sioux Valley Hospital
1100 South Euclid Avenue
P.O. Box 5039

Sioux Falls, SD
57117-5039
Yvonne Bailey, RN

Tennessee

Baptist Memorial Hospital
Medical Center
899 Madison Avenue
Memphis, TN 38146
Shelly Branch, RN

Donelson Hospital
The Diabetes Center
3055 Lebanon Road
Nashville, TN 37215
Catherine Tibbetts, BSN,
MPH

Endocrinology-Diabetes
Associates
Diabetes Care Program
4230 Harding Road, Suite
527
Nashville, TN 37205
Anne Brown, CDE, MSN

Erlanger Medical Center
Regional Diabetes Center
975 East Third Street
Chattanooga, TN 37403
Mary Goodner, RN, CDE

Indian Path Medical Center
Diabetes Treatment Centers
of America
2000 Brookside Road
Kingsport, TN 37660
Dayle C. Benson

*LeBonheur Children's
Medical Center
Diabetes Education
Program
One Children's Plaza
Memphis, TN 38103
Beverly West, RN, BSN,
CDE

Regional Medical Center at
Memphis
877 Jefferson Avenue
Memphis, TN 38103
Anna Averill, RN, CDE

Department of VA Medical
Center
Memphis VA Diabetes
Education Program
Memphis, TN 38104
Clyde Elder, RN, MSN,
CDE

University of Tennessee
Medical Center
The Diabetes Center
1924 Alcoa Highway
Knoxville, TN 37920
Catherine Thomas,
RN

Texas

AMI Park Plaza Hospital
Diabetes Treatment Centers
of America
1313 Herman Drive
Houston, TX 77004
Emily Cook, MEd

Baylor University Medical
  Center
Ruth Collins Diabetes
  Center
3500 Gaston Avenue
Dallas, TX 75246
Deborah K. Dennis, RN,
  BS, CDE

*Children's Diabetes
  Management Center
Department of Pediatrics
University of Texas
  Medical Branch
Galveston, TX 77550
Barbara Schreiner, RN,
  MN, CDE
Luther B. Travis, MD, CDE

Endocrine Associates of
  Dallas P.A.
5480 La Sierra Drive
Dallas, TX 75231
Joan Colgin, RN, BSN, CDE

High Plains Baptist Hospital
Center for Diabetes Care
1600 Wallace Blvd
Amarillo, TX 79106
Karen King, RN

Irving Hospital
Diabetes Lifestyle Center
1901 North MacArthur
Irving, TX 75061
Sally Hill, RN, CDE

St. David's Hospital
Diabetes Center

Box 4039
Austin, TX 78765-4039
Mary Hight

Scott & White Clinic
Diabetes Education
  Program
2401 S. 31st Street
Temple, TX 76508
Veronica Piziak, MD

Spohn Hospital
600 Elizabeth Street
Corpus Christi, TX 78404
Cheryl Jay, RN, BSN

Utah

HCA, St. Mark's Hospital
Diabetes Treatment Centers
  of America
1200 East 3900 South
Salt Lake City, UT 84124
Judy Loper

Holy Cross Hospital
Center for Diabetes
  Management and
  Research
1050 East South Temple
Salt Lake City, UT 84102
William Bruce

Virginia

Allegheny Regional
  Hospital
Diabetes Education Program
Exit 6, I-64

Low Moor, VA 24457
Brenda Lindsay, RN, BSN

Chippenham Medical
  Center
Diabetes Treatment Center
7101 Jahnke Road
Richmond, VA 23225

DePaul Medical Center
150 Kingsley Lane
Norfolk, VA 23505
Kathy Grillo, RN, MEd,
  CDE

Loudoun Healthcare, Inc.
Diabetes Management
  Program
224 Cornwall Street N.W.
Leesburg, VA 22075
Debbie Sauvé, MSN, RN,
  CDE

Richmond Diabetes
  Management Center
7301 Forest Avenue
Richmond, VA 23226
Sallie Bartholomew, RN,
  CDE

The Memorial Hospital
Diabetes Education
  Program
142 South Main Street
Danville, VA 24541
Lois Herb, RN

Fairfax Hospital
IDC-Virginia
3300 Gallows Road

Falls Church, VA 22046
Kathryn Mulcahy, RN

Jefferson Hospital
Diabetes Management
  Center
4600 King Street
Alexandria, VA 22302
Barbara Staiger, RN

Roanoke Memorial
  Hospitals
Diabetes Care Unit
Belleview at Jefferson Street
Roanoke, VA 24033
Flora Cantor, RN

Washington

St. Joseph Hospital and
  Health Care Center
Diabetes Education Program
1718 South I Street
P.O. Box 2197
Tacoma, WA 98401
Jacqueline Siegel, MN, RN,
  CDE

Virginia Mason Medical
  Center
Diabetes Center
1100 Ninth Avenue
Seattle, WA 98111

West Virginia

Camden-Clark Memorial
  Hospital
Diabetes Management
  Center

800 Garfield Avenue
P.O. Box 718
Parkersburg, WV 26101
Cherrie Cowan, RN, BSN,
  CDE

Wisconsin

*Children's Hospital of
  Wisconsin
9000 West Wisconsin
  Avenue
P.O. Box 1997
Milwaukee, WI 53201
Marian Benz, MS, RD,
  CDE

Columbia Hospital
Diabetes Treatment Centers
  of America
2025 East Newport
  Avenue
Milwaukee, WI 53211
Mark Klosiewski, RN,
  MSN, CDE

Dean Medical Center
Diabetes Program
1313 Fish Hatchery Road
Madison, WI 53715
Dory Blobner, RN, MS, CDE

Froedtert Memorial
  Lutheran Hospital

Diabetes Care Center
Medical College of
  Wisconsin
9200 W. Wisconsin
  Avenue
Milwaukee, WI 53226
Julie Kuenzi, RN, MSN,
  CDE

Prairie Clinic, S.C.
Diabetes Focus Program
55 Prairie Avenue
Prairie du Sac, WI 53578
Catherine M. Boatwright,
  RN, BSN

St. Luke's Medical Center
Diabetes Education
  Program
2900 W. Oklahoma
  Avenue
Milwaukee, WI 53215
Lois Salzwedel, RN, CDE

Wyoming

DePaul Hospital
Diabetes Education
  Program
2600 East 18th Street
Cheyenne, WY 82001
Amy Jaraczeski, RN, CDE

The following centers also provide diabetes care and education:

DIABETES TREATMENT CENTERS

Diabetes Treatment Centers of America
One Burton Hills Boulevard
Nashville, TN 37215
615-665-1133
Nation-wide treatment facilities located in traditional hospital settings. Many, but not all, offer in-patient education programs of a week's duration or more. (See expanded listings on page 168.)

Joslin Diabetes Center
One Joslin Place
Boston, MA 02215
617-732-2400
(See expanded listings on page 171.)
Affiliated with:

Memorial Medical Center
3627 University Boulevard
Jacksonville, FL 32216
904-391-1500
One of the first centers devoted exclusively to diabetes treatment. Also a research center.

Joslin Diabetes Clinic at St. Barnabas Medical Center
101 Old Short Hills Road
West Orange, NJ 07052
201-325-6555
Serving New York, New Jersey, and Pennsylvania.

Diabetes Treatment Unit–The New York Eye and Ear Infirmary
310 East 14th Street
New York, NY 10003
212-979-4000
Patients must be referred by their own physician. Emphasis is on self-care information. Regulation program has limited enrollment for its week-long in-patient setting.

International Diabetes Center–Park Nicollet Medical Foundation
500 West 39th Street
Minneapolis, MN 55416
612-927-3393
Has affiliates in other locations.
Not an in-patient program, but it does attract clients from throughout the country. IDC is a major education center for both patients
and health professionals, as well as a publisher of educational
materials.

DIABETES TREATMENT CENTERS OF AMERICA

Alexian Brothers Medical
Center
800 West Bietsterfield
Road
Elk Grove Village, IL 60007
312-981-5565

Baptist Medical Center
9601 Interstate 630, Exit 7
Little Rock, AR 72205-7299
501-227-1877

Children's Hospital of San
Francisco
3700 California Street
4 East
San Francisco, CA 94118
415-750-6506

Columbia Hospital
2025 East Newport Avenue
Milwaukee, WI 53211
414-961-4641

Cooper Hospital/University
Medical Center
One Cooper Plaza

Camden, NJ 08103
609-342-2939

Doctors Hospital of
Columbus
616 19th Street
Columbus, GA 31993
404-571-4161

Doctors Hospital of
Lakewood
3700 East South Street
Lakewood, CA 90712
213-408-0454

Erlanger Medical Center
975 East Third Street
Chattanooga, TN 37403
615-778-3939

Foothill Presbyterian
Hospital
250 South Grand Avenue
Glendora, CA 91740
818-914-1911
Mailing address:
150 South Grand Avenue

Suite B
Glendora, CA 91740

Georgetown University
  Hospital
3800 Reservoir Road N.W.
7 Bles, 7th floor
Washington, DC 20007
202-784-2200

Glendale Adventist
  Medical Center
1509 Wilson Terrace
Glendale, CA 91206
818-500-0256 x 7759

Holy Cross Hospital
1050 East South Temple
Salt Lake City, UT 84102
801-350-8114

Lee Memorial Hospital
2776 Cleveland Avenue
Fort Myers, FL 33902
813-334-5200

Mercy Hospital
3663 South Miami Avenue
Miami, FL 33133
305-285-2930

Mercy Hospital & Medical
  Center
Stevenson Expressway &
  King Drive
Chicago, IL 60616
312-567-8775

Methodist Hospital
580 West 8th Street

Jacksonville, FL 32209
904-798-8195

Metropolitan Hospital—
  Central
201 N. Eighth Street
Philadelphia, PA 19106
215-238-2951

Metropolitan Hospital—
  Parkview
1331 E. Wyoming Avenue
Philadelphia, PA 19124
215-537-7951

Metropolitan Hospital—
  Springfield
190 W. Sproul Road
Springfield, PA 19064
215-328-8951

Metropolitan Mt. Sinai
  Medical Center
900 South 8th Street
Minneapolis, MN 55404
612-347-4208

Monmouth Medical
  Center
300 Second Avenue
Long Branch, NJ 07740
201-870-5696

Montgomery Hospital
Powell & Fornance Streets
Norristown, PA 19401
215-270-2301

Moses Taylor Hospital
700 Quincy Avenue

Scranton, PA 18510
717-963-2140

Newark Beth Israel
    Medical Center
201 Lyons Avenue
Newark, NJ 07112
201-926-3218

Orlando Regional Medical
    Center
1414 South Kuhl Avenue
Orlando, FL 32806-2093
407-237-6330

AMI Park Plaza
    Hospital
1313 Hermann Drive
Houston, TX 77004
713-527-5761

HCA/Raleigh Community
    Hospital
3400 Old Wake Forest
    Road
Raleigh, NC 27609

RHD Memorial Medical
    Center
LBJ Freeway at Webbs
    Chapel Road
Dallas, TX 75381-9094
214-888-7005

Riverside Community
    Hospital
4445 Magnolia
    Avenue
Riverside, CA 92501
714-788-3491

Roper Hospital
316 Calhoun Street
Charleston, SC 29401-1125
803-724-2412

Rose Medical Center
4567 East 9th Avenue
Denver, CO 80220
303-320-2490

St. Joseph Medical Center
3600 East Harry Street
Wichita, KS 67218
316-689-6080

Somerset Medical Center
110 Rehill Avenue
Somerville, NJ 08876
201-685-2846

Sun Towers Hospital
1801 North Oregon Street
El Paso, TX 79902
915-533-7585

AMI Tarzana Regional
    Medical Center
18321 Clark Street
Tarzana, CA 91356
818-708-5455

Trinity Lutheran Hospital
3030 Baltimore
Kansas City, MO 64108
816-753-5100

United Hospital
333 North Smith Avenue
St. Paul, MN 55102
612-298-8780

University Community
  Hospital
3100 East Fletcher Avenue
Tampa, FL 33613
813-972-7262

Waltham Weston Hospital
  & Medical Center
5 Hope Avenue
Waltham, MA 02254-9116
617-647-6222

Wesley Long Community
  Hospital
501 North Elam Avenue
P.O. Box Drawer X-3
Greensboro, NC 27403
919-854-6142

Western Medical Center
1001 North Tustin Avenue
Santa Ana, CA 92705
714-953-3620

HCA/West Paces Ferry
  Hospital
3200 Howell Mill Road
  N.W.
Atlanta, GA 30327
404-350-5555

*JOSLIN DIABETES
  CENTERS*

Joslin Diabetes Clinic
Morton Plant Hospital
Clearwater, FL 34616
813-461-8300

Joslin Diabetes Clinic
Memorial Medical
  Center
Jacksonville, FL 32216
904-391-1500

Joslin Diabetes Clinic
Baptist Hospital of
  Miami
8900 N. Kendall Drive
Miami, FL 33176
800-992-1879

Joslin Diabetes Clinic
Methodist Hospital of
  Indiana and Diabetes
  and Endocrinology
  Associates
Indianapolis, IN 46260
317-843-0000

Joslin Diabetes
  Center
Boston, MA 02215
617-732-2400;
Framingham, MA 01701
508-620-9600

Joslin Diabetes Clinic
Saint Barnabas Medical
  Center
101 Old Short Hills Road
West Orange, NJ 07052
201-325-6555

Joslin Diabetes Clinic
West Penn Hospital
Pittsburgh, PA 15224
412-578-1724

JDF CHAPTERS

Birmingham Chapter
P.O. Box 360253
Birmingham, AL 35236
205-326-9995

First Arkansas Chapter
101 Fox Creek
Hot Springs, AR 71901
501-321-9182

Greater Phoenix Chapter
One East Camelback
Suite 605
Phoenix, AZ 85012
602-264-0370

Inland Empire Chapter
1520 N. Waterman Avenue
San Bernardino, CA 92404
714-888-3298

Los Angeles Chapter
10811 Washington Blvd.
Suite #301
Culver City, CA 90232
213-842-6742

Orange County Chapter
17200 Jamboree Blvd.
Suite K
Irvine, CA 92714
714-553-0363

Riverside Chapter
3526 Nelson Street
Riverside, CA 92506
909-369-1392

Sacramento Chapter
2151 River Plaza Drive,
   Suite 205
Sacramento, CA 95833
916-927-5676

San Diego Chapter
8304 Claremont Mass Blvd.
Suite #101
San Diego, CA 92111
619-279-9160

Greater Bay Area Chapter
1806 A Union Street
San Francisco, CA 94123
415-441-7720

Rocky Mountain Chapter
295 Clayton
Suite #204
Denver, CO 80206
303-321-7442

Colorado Springs Branch
719-684-2230

Greeley Chapter
P.O. Box 3134
Greeley, CO 80634
303-353-3602

Greater Hartford Chapter
18 North Main Street
West Hartford, CT 06107
203-561-1153

Greater New Haven
   Chapter
364 Whitney Avenue
New Haven, CT 06511
203-776-3200

Greater Hartford Chapter
18 North Main Street
Third Floor
West Hartford, CT 06107
203-561-1153

Fairfield County Chapter
4 Forest Street
New Canaan, CT 06840
203-972-1729

Greater Waterbury Guild
P.O. Box 788
Watertown, CT 06795
203-274-1407

First State Chapter
3202 Kirkwood Highway
Suite #206
Wilmington, DE 19808
302-633-3550

Capitol Chapter
1400 I Street N.W.
Suite #500
Washington, DC 20005
202-371-0044

Honolulu Chapter
826 Kainui Drive
Kailua, HI 96734
808-537-8312

South Florida Chapter
800 East Broward Blvd.
Suite #101
Fort Lauderdale, FL 33301
305-768-9008

Central Florida Chapter
266 Wilshire Blvd.
Suite #151
Casselberry, FL 32707
407-331-2873

Palm Beach Chapter
204 Brazilian Avenue
Suite #202
Palm Beach, FL 33480
407-655-0825

Greater Palm Beach County
  Chapter
6671 West Indiantown Rd.
Suite #56-347
Jupiter, FL 33458
405-840-0132

North Florida Guild
P.O. Box 56547
Jacksonville, FL 32241
904-260-2903

Tampa Bay Chapter
1 Progress Plaza
Suite #610
St. Petersburg, FL 33704
813-821-1616

Georgia Chapter
229 Peachtree St. N.E.
Caine Tower
Atlanta, GA 30303
404-688-2646

East Central Illinois
  Chapter
P.O. Box 192
Villa Grove, IL 61956
217-351-6997

Greater Chicago Chapter
70 W. Hubbard St. #205
Chicago, IL 60610
312-670-0313

Springfield Chapter
P.O. Box 2178
Springfield, IL 62705
217-787-7879

Greater Indianapolis
 Chapter
3011 Lucann Street
Carmel, IN 46033
317-844-2688

Southern Indiana Chapter
P.O. Box 53
Sullivan, IN 47882
812-382-4421

Central Iowa Chapter
P.O. Box 4644
Des Moines, IA 50306
515-967-6623

Northeast Iowa Chapter
602 Sycamore St.
Jamesville, IA 50647
319-987-2083

Kansas City Chapter
P.O. Box 6553
Shawnee Mission, KS
 66206
816-444-4688

Louisville Chapter
P.O. Box #6831
Louisville, KY 40206
502-566-6828

Campbellsville Chapter
418 Green Leaf Drive
Campbellsville, KY 42719
502-465-3154

Bluegrass Chapter
103 Robinson Drive
Richmond, KY 40475
606-624-2637

Louisiana Chapter
3456 Cleary Avenue
Suite #602
Metairie, LA 70002
504-887-1600

Portland Chapter
P.O. Box 426
Westbrook, ME 04092
207-854-8710

Central Maryland Chapter
5 E. Gwynn Mills Court
Owing Mills, MD 21117
410-356-4555

Worcester County Chapter
45 Timrod Drive
Worcester, MA 01603
508-753-0742

Bay State Chapter
770 Dedham Street
Canton, MA 02021
617-575-0677

Greater Springfield Chapter
11 Acorn Lane
Ludlow, MA 01054
413-589-0687

Metropolitan Detroit
  Chapter
29350 Southfield Road
  #114
Southfield, MI 48076
313-569-6171

Ann Arbor Branch
313-662-4708

S.W. Suburban Detroit
  Branch
15544 Michigan Avenue
Dearborn, MI 48126
313-582-7520

Upper Peninsula Chapter
85 1st Street
Laurium, MI 49913
906-337-5928

West Michigan Chapter
4362 Cascade Road S.E.
Suite # 116
Grand Rapids, MI 49546
616-957-1838

Hiawathaland Chapter
P.O. Box 6953
Rochester, MN 55903
507-288-7847

Minneapolis/St. Paul
  Chapter
Butler North Bldg
510 1st Ave., No.
Suite #410
Minneapolis, MN 55403
612-455-0201

Southern Mississippi
  Chapter
Rte. 5, Box 511
Brookhaven, MS 39601
601-366-4400

St. Louis Chapter
225 South Meramec Ave.
Suite #400
Clayton MO 63105
314-726-6778

Lincoln Chapter
P.O. Box 94625
Lincoln, NE 68509
402-467-2254

Omaha Council Bluffs
  Chapter
P.O. Box 241209
Omaha, NE 68124
402-592-3948

Las Vegas Chapter
4220 South Maryland
  Parkway, Suite #112
Las Vegas, NV 89119
702-732-4795

New Hampshire Chapter
P.O. Box 3194
Nashua, NH 03061
603-595-2595

Cape Atlantic Chapter
c/o Argus Real Estate
6511 Ventnor Ave
Atlantic City, NJ 08406
609-823-0689

Central Jersey Chapter
146 Maple Avenue
Red Bank, NJ 07701
908-842-8117

North Jersey Chapter
513 W. Mt. Pleasant Ave.
Livingston, NJ 07039
201-992-0375

Princeton Guild
72 Arreton Road
Princeton, NJ 08540
609-497-2060

South Jersey Chapter
496 Kings Highway North
Cherry Hill, NJ 08034
609-779-9202

Tri-County Chapter
139 Raritan Avenue
Highland Park, NJ 08904
201-249-1711

Albuquerque Chapter
P.O. Box 35388
Albuquerque, NM 87176
505-883-9532

Binghamton Chapter
46 Felters Road
Binghamton, NY 13903
607-772-1728

Dutchess County Chapter
Eclison Motor Inn
Route 55
Poughkeepsie, NY 12603
914-454-9458

Long Island/South Shore
    Chapter
P.O. Box 358
Cedarhurst, NY 11516
516-569-2200

MidHudson Chapter
P.O. Box 352
Westtown, NY 10998
914-355-1625

Nassau-Suffolk
    Chapter
350 Willis Avenue
Mineola, NY 11501
516-739-2873

Westchester Branch
914-238-3949

New York Chapter
381 Park Ave. South
Suite #507
New York, NY 10016
212-689-2860

Brooklyn, NY Branch
718-768-0095

Staten Island, NY
    Branch
718-727-5325

Queens, NY Branch
718-478-1594

Rockland/Bergen/Passaic
    Chapter
0-108 29th Street
Fair Lawn, NJ 07410
201-791-7155

Capital-Saratoga
  Chapter
26 Twilight Drive
Clifton Park, NY 12065
518-449-1360

Syracuse Chapter
Box 71 Solvay Station
Syracuse, NY 13209
315-474-0601

Ulster County Chapter
P.O. Box 24
Lake Katrine, NY 12449
914-336-5426

Western New York
  Chapter
442 Beach Road at
  Maryvale
Buffalo, NY 14225
716-632-2873

Asheville Guild
5 Arboretum Road
Asheville, NC 28803
704-274-3136

Blue Ridge Chapter
1114 Little John Drive
Morganton, NC 28655
704-728-8466

Charlotte Chapter
1012 South King Drive
Suite #701
Charlotte, NC 28283
704-377-2873

N.E. North Carolina Chapter
1812½ N Road
Elizabeth City, NC 27909
919-335-0107

Central Carolina Chapter
P.O. Box 14393
Research Triangle Park, NC
  27709
919-775-3821

Greater Cincinnati Chapter
10901 Reed Hartman Hway.
Suite #202
Cincinnati, OH 45242
513-793-3223

Cleveland Chapter
4500 Rockside Road
Suite #420
Cleveland, OH 44131
216-524-6000

Greater Dayton Chapter
4610 Penn Avenue
Suite #302
Dayton, OH 45458
513-256-2873

Mid-Ohio Chapter
1700 Arlingate Lane
Columbus, OH 43228
614-278-2474

East Central Ohio Chapter
4510 Belden Village St.
  N.W.
Suite #L-15
Canton, OH 44718
216-492-2873

Northwest Ohio Chapter
5241 Southwyck Blvd.
Suite #220
Toledo, OH 43614
419-866-8878

Central Oklahoma Chapter
P.O. Box 636
Norman, OK 73070
405-364-1583

Greater Portland Chapter
1281 Overlook Drive
Lake Oswego, OR 97034
503-638-8825

Greater ABE Chapter
539 North 16th Street
Allentown, PA 18102
215-820-0125

Berks County Chapter
1213 Lancaster Park West
Reading, PA 19607
215-775-4169

Greater Harrisburg Chapter
2600 North Third Street
Harrisburg, PA 17110
717-233-6855

Lawrence County Chapter
RD 6 Box 319
New Castle, PA 16101
412-924-2941

Norristown Chapter
5108 Brandywine Drive
Eagleville, PA 19403
215-630-1490

Philadelphia Chapter
2200 Benjamin Franklin
   Parkway
Philadelphia, PA 19130
215-567-5334

Greater Pittsburgh
   Chapter
300 Sixth Avenue
Suite #273
Pittsburgh, PA 15222
412-471-1414

Low Country Chapter
667 Ferry Street
Mt. Pleasant, SC 29464
803-766-0385

Palmetto Chapter
3608 Landmark Drive,
   Suite C
Columbia, SC 29204
803-782-1477

Sioux Falls Chapter
P.O. Box 88540
Sioux Falls, SD
   57104-8540
605-338-2295

Watertown Chapter
107 Summerwood Drive
Watertown, SD 57201
605-886-5173

East Tennessee Chapter
401 Philpott Drive–RT 3
Box 30460
Madisonville, TN 37354
615-442-3861

Greater Knoxville Chapter
P.O. Box 566
Knoxville, TN 37920
615-577-7530

Central Tennessee Chapter
2400 Crestmoor
Nashville, TN 37215
615-386-7188

Abilene Chapter
P.O. Box 6054
Abilene, TX 79608
915-675-6046

Dallas Chapter
9400 N. Central
    Expressway
Suite #9
Dallas, TX 75231
214-373-9808

Houston Gulf Coast
    Chapter
5075 Westheimer
Suite #682
Houston, TX 77056
713-965-9742

West Texas Chapter
P.O. Box 7308
Midland, TX 79708
915-684-0902

South Central Chapter
4115 Medical Drive
Suite #202
San Antonio, TX 78229
512-692-9264

Salt Lake City Chapter
158 East 100 North
Farmington, UT 84025
801-451-5682

Greater Lynchburg Chapter
105 Crestline Drive
Forest, VA 24551
804-525-2462

Roanoke Valley Chapter
3201 Brandon Avenue
    S.W.
Suite #5
Roanoke, VA 24018
703-989-6627

Southside VA Chapter
725 Tuscarora Drive
Danville, VA 24540
804-793-4133

Seattle Chapter
Tillicum Marina
1333 N. Northlake Way
Suite #G
Seattle, WA 98103
206-545-1510

Seattle Guild
1001 4th Avenue
Suite #4725
Seattle, WA 98154
206-343-0873

Spokane County Area
    Chapter
P.O. Box 3705
Spokane, WA 99220
509-458-4437

Huntington Chapter
P.O. Box 2903
Huntington, WV 25728
304-523-4533

Fox Valley Chapter
P.O. Box 101
Appleton, WI 54914
414-738-6788

Greater Madison
  Chapter
P.O. Box 1347
Madison, WI 53701
608-836-4408

Milwaukee Chapter
2323 North Mayfair
  Road
Wauwatosa, WI 53226
414-453-4673

JDF AFFILIATES

Juvenile Diabetes
  Foundation Canada

JDF Canada
89 Granton Drive
Richmond Hill, Ontario
L4B 2N5
1-416-889-4171

Burlington/Hamilton
  Chapter
3040 New Street
2nd Floor, Suite 4

Burlington, Ontario
L7N 1M5
1-416-333-4660

Calgary Chapter
5920–1A Street S.W.
Suite 417
Calgary, Alberta
T2H 0G3
1-403-255-7100

Edmonton Chapter
9924–106 Street
Suite 202
Edmonton, Alberta
T5K 1C4
1-403-428-0343

Montreal Chapter
3767 Thimens Blvd.
Suite 260
St. Laurent, Quebec
H4R 1W4
1-514-339-1983
1-800-361-1278

Red Deer Chapter
#223, 3722–57th
  Avenue
Red Deer, Alberta
T4N 4R6
1-403-347-0070

Perth Chapter
c/o Garry Turnbull
R.R. #7, P.O. Box 214
Perth, Ontario
K7H 3E3
1-613-264-0456

Ottawa Chapter
1129 Carling Avenue
Ottawa, Ontario
K1Y 4G6
1-613-729-8760

Regina Chapter
P.O. Box 3924
Regina, Saskatchewan
S4P 3R8
1-306-789-8474

Saskatoon Chapter
2nd Floor 233-22nd Street E.
Saskatoon, Saskatchewan
S7K 0G3
1-306-244-5335

Toronto Chapter
49 The Donway West
Suite 320
Don Mills, Ontario
M3C 3M9
1-416-510-1350

Vancouver Chapter
#5, 1496 West 72nd
  Avenue
Vancouver, British
  Columbia
V6P 3C8

Region of Waterloo
  Chapter
P.O. Box 71
Station C
Kitchener, Ontario
N2G 3W9
1-519-745-2426

Winnipeg Chapter
900 St. James Street
#208
Winnipeg, Manitoba
R3G 3J7
1-204-775-7928

JDF Australia
P.O. Box 1500
Chatswood NSW 2057,
  Australia
61-02-411-4087

AJD Brazil
Rua Batatais, 602
  #6462
Sao Paulo 01423, Brazil
55-11-284-4302

JDF Chile
Est. Metro Esc.
Militar, Gal. Sur, Lc. 12
Las Condes
Santiago, Chile
56-2-2288646

JDF United Kingdom
25 Gosfield Street
London, England W1P
  7HB
44-71-436-3112

DSJ France
8, rue du Temple
Cognac 16100, France
011-33-45-82-5404

JDF Hellas
47 Vasilissis Sofias Ave.

Athens 10676, Greece
30-1-7225828

JDF Calcutta
800 H Lake Town
Calcutta 700089, India

JDF Israel
5 Jabotinsky Street
Tel Aviv 63479, Israel
972-3-546-3830

JDF Italia
Via Regina Margherita, 42
00198 Roma, Italy
39-6-8455041

JDF Puerto Rico
P.O. Box 70137
San Juan, Puerto Rico
   00936
809-751-6641

ABOUT THE AUTHORS

Woody and Sale Johnson have been active in diabetes-related causes since their daughter Casey was diagnosed as diabetic when she was eight. Woody, who has testified before Congress and the NIH, is currently co-chairman of the Juvenile Diabetes Foundation's $100 million fund-raising initiative, and Sale has chaired several related events. Casey is a student at the Marymount School in New York City, where she lives with her parents and her younger sisters, Jaime and Daisy.

Susan Kleinman is a freelance journalist and speechwriter based in New York City. She writes frequently on health and family issues, and is the author of *Real Life 101: Almost Surviving Your First Year Out of College* (MasterMedia, 1989) and a revised edition, for these turbulent times, titled *Real Life 101: The Graduate's Guide to Survival* (MasterMedia, May 1992). She is co-author of *The Big Apple Business and Pleasure Guide.*

Additional copies of *Managing Your Child's Diabetes* may be ordered by sending a check for $10.95 for the paperback edition or $18.95 for the cloth edition (please add the following for postage and handling: $2.00 for the first copy, $1.00 for each additional copy) to:

MasterMedia Limited
17 East 89th Street
New York, NY 10128

(212)260-5600
(800)334-8232
(212)348-2020 (fax)

The Johnsons and Susan Kleinman are available for keynotes and seminars. Please contact MasterMedia's Speakers' Bureau for availability and fee arrangements. Call Tony Colao at (908)359-1612 or (908)359-1647 (fax).

OTHER MASTERMEDIA BOOKS

THE PREGNANCY AND MOTHERHOOD DIARY: Planning the First Year of Your Second Career, by Susan Schiffer Stautberg, is the first and only undated appointment diary that shows how to manage pregnancy and career. ($12.95 spiralbound)

CITIES OF OPPORTUNITY: Finding the Best Place to Work, Live and Prosper in the 1990's and Beyond, by Dr. John Tepper Marlin, explores the job and living options for the next decade and into the next century. This consumer guide and handbook, written by one of the world's experts on cities, selects and features forty-six American cities and metropolitan areas. ($13.95 paper, $24.95 cloth)

THE DOLLARS AND SENSE OF DIVORCE: The Financial Guide for Women, by Judith Briles, is the first book to combine practical tips on overcoming the legal hurdles with planning before, during and after divorce ($10.95 paper)

OUT THE ORGANIZATION: New Career Opportunities for the 1990s, by Robert and Madeleine Swain, is written for the millions of Americans whose jobs are no longer safe, whose companies are not loyal and who face futures of uncertainty. It gives advice on finding a new job or starting your own business. ($12.95 paper, $17.95 cloth)

185

AGING PARENTS AND YOU: A Complete Handbook to Help You Help Your Elders Maintain a Healthy, Productive and Independent Life, by Eugenia Anderson-Ellis and Marsha Dryan, is a complete guide to providing care to aging relatives. It gives practical advice and resources to the adults who are helping their elders lead productive and independent lives. ($9.95 paper)

CRITICISM IN YOUR LIFE: How to Give It, How to Take It, How to Make It Work for You, by Dr. Deborah Bright, offers practical advice, in an upbeat, readable and realistic fashion, for turning criticism into control. Charts and diagrams guide the reader into managing criticism from bosses, spouses, children, friends, neighbors and in-laws. ($9.95 paper, $17.95 cloth)

BEYOND SUCCESS: How Volunteer Service Can Help You Begin Making a Life Instead of Just a Living, by John F. Raynolds III and Eleanor Raynolds, C.B.E., is a unique how-to book targeted to business and professional people considering volunteer work, senior citizens who wish to fill leisure time meaningfully and students trying out various career options. The book is filled with interviews with celebrities, CEOs and average citizens who talk about the benefits of service work. ($9.95 paper, $19.95 cloth)

MANAGING IT ALL: Time-Saving Ideas for Career, Family, Relationships and Self, by Beverly Benz Treuille and Susan Schiffer Stautberg, is written for women who are juggling careers and families. Over two hundred career women (ranging from a TV anchorwoman to an investment banker) were interviewed. The book contains many humorous anecdotes on saving time and improving the quality of life for self and family. ($9.95 paper)

REAL LIFE 101: The Graduate's Guide to Survival, by Susan Kleinman, supplies welcome advice to those facing "real life" for the first time, focusing on work, money, health and how to deal with freedom and responsibility. ($9.95 paper)

YOUR HEALTHY BODY, YOUR HEALTHY LIFE: How to Take Control of Your Medical Destiny, by Donald B. Louria, M.A., provides precise advice and strategies that will help you to live a long and healthy life. Learn also about nutrition, exercise, vitamins and medication, as well as how to control risk factors for major diseases. ($12.95 paper)

THE CONFIDENCE FACTOR: How Self-Esteem Can Change Your Life, by Judith Briles, is based on a nationwide survey of six thousand men and women. Briles explores why women so often feel a lack of self-confidence and have a poor opinion of themselves. She offers step-by-step advice on becoming the person you want to be. ($9.95 paper, $18.95 cloth)

THE SOLUTION TO POLLUTION: 101 Things You Can Do to Clean Up Your Environment, by Laurence Sombke, offers step-by-step techniques on how to conserve more energy, start a recycling center, choose biodegradable products and proceed with individual environmental cleanup projects. ($7.95 paper)

TAKING CONTROL OF YOUR LIFE: The Secrets of Successful Enterprising Women, by Gail Blanke and Kathleen

Walas, is based on the authors' professional experience with Avon Products' Women of Enterprise Awards, given each year to outstanding women entrepreneurs. The authors offer a specific plan to help you gain control over your life and include business tips and quizzes as well as beauty and lifestyle information. ($17.95 cloth)

SIDE-BY-SIDE STRATEGIES: How Two-Career Couples Can Thrive in the Nineties, by Jane Hershey Cuozzo and S. Diane Graham, describes how two-career couples can learn the difference between competing with a spouse and becoming a supportive power partner. Published in hardcover as *Power Partners.* ($10.95 paper, $19.95 cloth)

DARE TO CONFRONT! How to Intervene When Someone You Care About Has an Alcohol or Drug Problem, by Bob Wright and Deborah George Wright, shows the reader how to use the step-by-step methods of professional intervention-ists to motivate drug-dependent people to accept the help they need. ($17.95 cloth)

WORK WITH ME! How to Make the Most of Office Support Staff, by Betsy Lazary, shows how to find, train, and nurture the "perfect" assistant and how best to utilize your support staff professionals. ($9.95 paper)

MANN FOR ALL SEASONS: Wit and Wisdom from The Washington Post's *Judy Mann,* by Judy Mann, shows the columnist at her best as she writes about women, families and the politics of the women's revolution. ($9.95 paper, $19.95 cloth)

THE SOLUTION TO POLLUTION IN THE WORKPLACE, by Laurence Sombke, Terry M. Robertson and Elliot M. Kaplan, supplies employees with everything they need to know about cleaning up their workspace, including recycling, using energy efficiently, conserving water and buying recycled products and nontoxic supplies. ($9.95 paper)

THE ENVIRONMENTAL GARDENER: The Solution to Pollution for Lawns and Gardens, by Laurence Sombke, focuses on what each of us can do to protect our endangered plant life. A practical sourcebook and shopping guide. ($8.95 paper)

THE LOYALTY FACTOR: Building Trust in Today's Workplace, by Carol Kinsey Goman, Ph.D., offers techniques for restoring commitment and loyalty in the workplace. ($9.95 paper)

DARE TO CHANGE YOUR JOB—AND YOUR LIFE, by Carole Kanchier, Ph.D., provides a look at career growth and development throughout the life cycle. ($10.95 paper)

MISS AMERICA: In Pursuit of the Crown, by Ann-Marie Bivans, is an authorized guidebook to the Pageant, containing eyewitness accounts, complete historical data, and a realistic look at the trials and triumphs of potential Miss Americas. ($27.50 cloth)

POSITIVELY OUTRAGEOUS SERVICE: New and Easy Ways to Win Customers for Life, by T. Scott Gross, identifies what the consumers of the nineties really want and how businesses can develop effective marketing strategies to answer those needs. ($14.95 paper)

BREATHING SPACE: Living and Working at a Comfortable Pace in a Sped-Up Society, by Jeff Davidson, helps readers to handle information and activity overload and gain greater control over their lives. ($10.95 paper)

TWENTYSOMETHING: Managing and Motivating Today's New Work Force, by Lawrence J. Bradford, Ph.D., and Claire Raines, M.A., examines the work orientation of the younger generation, offering managers in businesses of all kinds a practical guide to better understand and supervise their young employees. ($22.95 cloth)

BALANCING ACTS! Juggling Love, Work, Family and Recreation, by Susan Schiffer Stautberg and Marcia L. Worthing, provides strategies to achieve a balanced life by reordering priorities and setting realistic goals. ($12.95 paper)

THE LIVING HEART BRAND NAME SHOPPER'S GUIDE, by Michael E. DeBakey, M.D., Antonio M. Gotto, Jr., M.D., D.Phil., Lynne W. Scott, M.A., R.D./L.D., and John P. Foreyt, Ph.D., lists brand name supermarket products that are low in fat, saturated fatty acids, and cholesterol. ($12.50 paper)

REAL BEAUTY . . . REAL WOMEN: A Workbook for Making the Best of Your Own Good Looks, by Kathleen Walas, National Beauty and Fashion Director of Avon Products, offers expert advice on beauty and fashion to women of all ages and ethnic backgrounds. ($19.50 cloth)

STEP FORWARD: Sexual Harassment in the Workplace, by Susan L. Webb, teaches the reader all the basic facts about sexual harassment and furnishes procedures to help stop it. ($9.95 paper)

INDEX